Melan

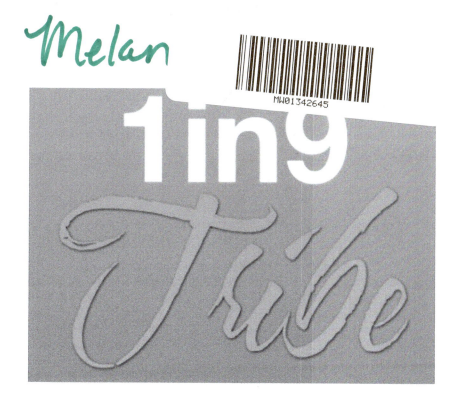

Kidney Disease Warriors Beating the
Drum of Hope and Change

Compiled by Analyn and Raymond Scott

Thank you for helping to amplify the sound of our drum!

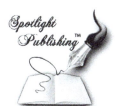

Spotlight Publishing
Goodyear, AZ

Analyn Scott

1in9 Tribe - Kidney Disease Warriors Beating the Drum of Hope and Change
© Copyright Analyn and Raymond Scott - 2019 First Edition

Part 8 used with permission from Microvascular Health Solutions and © 2019 Microvascular Health Solutions

ISBN: 978-1-7337388-0-4
ISBN: 978-1-7337388-1-1
Library of Congress Cataloging-in-Publication Data:

All rights reserved. No part of this book may be reproduced or transmitted in any form or by any means, electronic or mechanical, including photocopying, recording, or by any information storage and retrieval system, (electronic, mechanical, photocopying, recording or otherwise) without the prior written permission of the publisher. This book is sold subject to the condition that it shall not, by way of trade or otherwise, be lent, resold, hired out, or otherwise circulated without the publisher's prior consent in any form of binding or cover other than that in which it is published and without a similar condition, including this condition being imposed on the subsequent purchaser.

Editor: Becky Norwood
Cover: Angie Anyla - Fiverr.com/pro_ebookcovers
Interior Layout: ipublicidades.com

Disclaimer: ALL INFORMATION CONTAINED in this book and e-book is intended for your general knowledge only and is not a substitute for medical advice or treatment for specific medical conditions. I cannot and do not give you medical advice. If you have any specific questions about any medical matter, you should consult your doctor or a qualified professional healthcare provider. If you think you may be suffering from any medical condition you should seek immediate medical attention.

- Analyn and Raymond Scott
1in9 Tribe – Kidney Disease Warriors Beating the Drum of Hope and Change
Email: support@1in9KidneyChallenge.com
Website: www.1in9Tribe.com

Table of Contents

Special Message from 1in9 Founders –
Analyn and Raymond Scott 5

Part 1: We are 1in9 7

   Dance with Destiny - Analyn Scott 9
   My Hero - Kenyon Scott 21
   Stay Strong - Brooklyn Scott 25
   My Fight - Raymond Scott..29

Part 2: You are a Survivor!...33

   Paradigm Shift - Analyn Scott 35
   Reflections on Kidney Disease - Marilyn Brown Coleman 39
   What I Didn't Know Did Hurt Me - Isaac Johnson......................41
   This is My Story - Steve Harris 45
   The Prayer Jar - Shellisa Multrie 53

Part 3: Out of the Shadows..65

   "The Funky Diabetic" - Analyn Scott.......................................67
   A Legacy of Change - Micaiah & Micah Thomas.........................71
   My YES! - Josiah "Jojo" Martin 81

Part 4: It Takes a Village..87

   Babe & Bulldog - Analyn Scott...89
   Crowned for Change - Lisa Hedin..93
   Slow it Down CKD - Gail Rae-Garwood 103
   Faith and Basketball - Ericka Downey 115

Part 5: Medical Tribe **123**
    Vantage Point: A Nephrologist's View of
        Kidney Disease - Elise J. Barney, DO 125
    Helping Patients Thrive from Home - Dr. Sachin Desai 137
    Bank on Me - Dr. Jean Robey 143
    I Am Not My Disease - Raymond Scott 151

Part 6: The Drumbeat for Regenerative Medicine **155**
    The Future is NOW - Analyn Scott 157

Part 7: The Wheels of Change **163**
    Dialysis and Me - Maryjane Hamilton 165
    Pioneering the Future - Elizabeth Saladin, MD 185
    On the Road with 1in9 - Analyn Scott 191

Part 8: Getting to the Root **195**
    Discover Your Microvascular Health.
        Improve Your Future - Gary Hennerberg 197
    A Gift from Heaven - Analyn Scott 229

Part 9: Lift Up Your Voice **237**
    Amplify the Sound of Change 239
    "The 1in9" - Zemill 241

Special Message from 1in9 Founders

Analyn & Raymond Scott

As we celebrate 21 years of life since Raymond's kidneys failed, we reflect on the knowledge gained through our own experiences and from picking up the torch of advocacy and realize that it is time to challenge the status quo and bring kidney disease out of the public shadows of silence and misunderstanding to confront it head-on.

We are grateful for our "Tribe," those who have been with us from the beginning or through seasons of our journey. Our hearts are full of gratitude for our "1in9 Tribe" Warriors/co-authors who have lent their voices and impactful stories to help beat the drum of awareness and shatter the silence.

PART 1:

We Are 1in9

Dance with Destiny

Analyn Scott

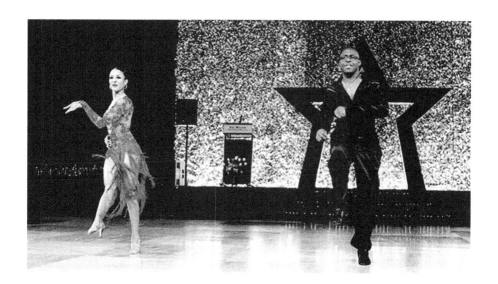

The time had finally arrived, and my heart was beating with great anticipation and pride as my husband Raymond was about to step out on the dance floor. It was February 20, 2016, and the Westin Kierland ballroom was transformed into a "Night of a Thousand Stars." As the unmistakable beat of Pharrell Williams' song "Happy" began, the spotlight, camera's, and all eyes were fixed on Raymond, and his professional dance instructor and partner, Briana. Their upbeat contagious energy spread throughout the room, as their choreographed steps moved to the beat, emphasizing the song's lyrics.

It was so much more than the six months of grueling dance lessons that prepared Raymond for this moment as one of the Celebrity Star Dancers at the 10th Annual Dancing with the Stars

Arizona competition, and fundraising gala hosted by the National Kidney Foundation of Arizona.

Let me take you back 18 years earlier where the journey to get here began. February 20, 1998, fell on a Friday. Raymond and I had been dating for three months, and we had plans that evening to go to dinner and a movie. He just had to go to urgent care that afternoon, thinking that he would get some antibiotics for a cough that had been bothering him for a week. He would call me a few hours later from the hospital with the shocking news that his kidneys had failed.

I can imagine the look on the nurse's face at the urgent care as she was taking his vital signs. Overall, Raymond was feeling ok, except for that awful cough and bout of nausea he had earlier in the week. He recounted to me how her eyes got big at the first blood pressure reading and how she took it two more times before running out of the room to get the doctor. 270/190 was the reading.

By the time the ambulance got him to the hospital emergency room, it was 300/200. "Mr. Scott, didn't you have a headache?" Asked the doctor, "You could have had a stroke. Didn't you have chest pain? You could have had a heart attack." His response was, "No, I just had this bad cough that I thought may have turned into bronchitis." He was partially right, he did have bronchitis, but that was the 10th diagnosis on the list. 1 through 9 are as follows:

1. Newly diagnosed end-stage renal disease secondary to hypertensive nephrosclerosis
2. Acute renal failure
3. Malignant hypertension
4. Electrolyte imbalance and hyponatremia, multifactorial
5. Acute and chronic failure
6. End-stage congestive heart failure

7. Hypertension
8. End-stage renal failure
9. Mitral valve disorder

Not the diagnosis you would expect for a 29-year-old who had just left the Army a year earlier is it? It wasn't what we expected or would have guessed either. Raymond's high blood pressure was triggered at the age of 22 after a bad car accident he was in, while in the military. Neither one of us knew that hypertension/high blood pressure was the second leading cause of kidney disease, nor that both were silent diseases. Had he better understood how interconnected they truly are, he would have been more proactive. Instead, when he left the military, he continued to take his blood pressure medications, and since he felt fine, he wasn't monitoring his blood pressures regularly.

This was the starting point of Raymond's dialysis journey.

Raymond was quiet for most of the ride home a week later when he was released from the hospital. I remember him turning to me and saying that he was going to move back home to Charleston, SC. "Why?" I asked. His reply was, "because I have a long road ahead of me and you're too young, and it wouldn't be fair to you." I was 23 at the time but quickly replied, "you're a good man, and you don't need to go anywhere. I'm not going to leave you because your kidneys failed, let's see where our relationship goes from here." A look of relief came across his face as he said, "I hoped you would say that, but I had to give you an out." Eleven months later we were married.

Over the years we've learned that Kidney disease and End-Stage Renal Disease (ESRD) don't follow a straight-line trajectory, but we continue to link arms and continue to take a step forward together at every twist and turn. More often than not, we had to learn through our experiences rather than being forewarned or prepared.

Raymond started on peritoneal dialysis (which will be better explained later in the book). This modality gave him more freedom because he could do his dialysis exchanges at home and work. With prior planning to ship his supplies, we were even able to take a cruise for our honeymoon. We were enjoying married life, I had started a new career in IT Sales, and we bought our first home. By this time, after about 2 or 2.5 years on this modality, it stopped working for him, and he began in-center hemodialysis. Oh my, what a huge difference, and not in a good way. He was exhausted and was thirsty all the time because his fluid intake was much more restricted since he was only getting dialysis treatments three days a week. Family members had offered before, but now Raymond was willing to have them be tested to donate a kidney. Without any hesitation, his younger brother Rome, who was stationed with the Marines in CA, offered to get tested. What a blessing and an immeasurable gift that he was able to donate a kidney to Raymond in October of 2001.

That's when we began trying to start a family. Getting pregnant was not as easy as we thought. After two rounds of IVF we welcomed our son Kenyon into this world in December 2004, moved into a new home in a better neighborhood, and we settled into a pretty typical family routine until the transplanted kidney failed in 2006 and Raymond had to go back to in-center hemodialysis. Raymond would rest as much as he could to build up enough energy to keep up with our happy, energetic son.

Raymond was on the transplant list, but without any calls, I decided to get tested to donate one of my kidneys to him in the summer of 2007...and, guess what, I was a match!!! We were excited to hear that the transplant would take place that October. Out of the blue, Raymond became extremely anemic and required several blood transfusions. A few weeks later we would get the call that because of the transfusions Raymond developed antibodies against me, and

I was no longer a match. Now for those that know me, you know I'm quite "determined," but I honestly took the news with stride thinking that God must not have wanted me to donate, and had other plans, so we both kept a positive outlook as we continued to move forward.

The Sunday before Thanksgiving 2007, Raymond called me from his dialysis center and said he was having difficulty breathing, so he was headed to the hospital. I was able to get Kenyon secured with my sister and was on my way to meet him there. Oxygen levels were low and being a dialysis patient; he was cared for fairly quickly. I remember there were several doctors in the room trying to figure out why he still had excess fluid when he had just finished dialyzing. Chest X-ray, EKG, and other tests were ordered, and it was determined that he had a pulmonary embolism - which later turned out to be a blessing in disguise. That's when I kicked into bulldog mode and ran down Raymond's medical history letting them know that Raymond has a high tolerance and doesn't always present with typical symptoms. The team decided to dialyze him again to remove the excess fluid, and the plan was to release him the next day.

I'll never forget the call I received from Raymond the next afternoon as I was pumping gas on my way to pick up Kenyon from my sister's house. He said, "Babe, they did an echocardiogram and found a tear in my heart, and I need to go in for emergency open heart surgery. I'm going to put the Cardiologist on the phone to explain more."

I remained strong and let Raymond know I would be there and was on my way. Then I listened to the doctor as he calmly explained that he needed me to sign some consent forms, and to drive safely, but to come now. It was as if I was walking in slow motion on air, you know, like in every Spike Lee movie. I got back in the van and started praying and making phone calls as I was driving. Our family is accustomed to my calling to keep them informed when Raymond had an issue, but what they were not used to was hearing or seeing me cry. My sister-n-law could immediately hear in my voice that something was wrong, and that's when the tears were released. I asked her to call their brothers. A wave of strength came over me, and I was able to restore my composure to tell my sister and Kenyon that he would need to stay there a few more days, then call the rest of my family members and my friend Kim. I made it safely and in record time to sign the consent forms, kiss Raymond and tell him I loved him, and that if he saw a bright light to go the other way! He promised me this, as he was wheeled off.

I was not alone as I sat in the waiting room for the next 6 or 7 hours. I can't emphasize enough the importance of having a strong support system when dealing with any chronic illness (as an individual or as a family). I'm eternally grateful for my beautifully diverse and loving tribe made up of family, chosen family and friends, not just that night, but throughout the twenty-one plus years of this journey. My mom, dad, and brother were able to get there before Raymond went into surgery. Kim and her mom Annette, who is a second mom to us, arrived with a book for me to read and a calming spirit and reassurance that Raymond was going to be ok.

Raymond had an elite Cardiology team on the case, which was needed since Raymond tends to keep things interesting. One of the cardiothoracic surgeons came out and informed us that the surgery was a success. They did an aortic arch graft replacement for the aortic dissection (an aortic aneurysm) and had to put in a mechanical heart valve. He explained how the elevated blood pressures had worn down the lining of Raymond's aorta over time, and he believed that Raymond probably had a small tear for over a month, but the pulmonary embolism widened the tear enough to cause the symptoms for him to come to the hospital before it ruptured.

To say that the first week was rough would be an understatement, but Raymond was receiving excellent care and was improving day by day. He was in the hospital for two weeks, and a little down because he couldn't come home in time for Kenyon's 3rd birthday party. I was able to brighten his spirits by telling him that I was pregnant! No IVF this time! God knew that had I given Raymond a kidney a month earlier his heart wouldn't have been able to take it, and we also wouldn't have our beautiful daughter Brooklyn.

As the primary breadwinner, I had to return to work, but thankfully my Uncle Blake had vacation time and welcomed the break to leave the Idaho snow for some Arizona sun. What a blessing and a relief it was to have him here to help make Raymond meals, drive him to and from dialysis and care for him during the day, and help me with Kenyon in the evenings. It was an act of love and service that we will never forget.

2008 was a rebound year. Raymond would continue with his in-center dialysis routine three days a week. In March I organized a surprise party to celebrate Raymond's 40th Birthday…with tons of help from my Tribe! We even had family fly in from Charleston to surprise him. They were shocked to see Raymond so thin. It's funny; I remember thinking that he needed to put more weight back on to look healthy. More on that later. Brooklyn was born in July, bringing more joy, love, and excitement to our family. Life was good.

I should point out that people on dialysis and those who have had a transplant have a weakened immune system, so we quickly learned that whenever Raymond gets a fever over 100, we take him to the emergency room. That protocol has made a critical difference on more than one occasion. During one of Raymond's many hospital visits, I remember Dr. Dahl, one of the Nephrologists with AKDHC that was on call, mentioning that Raymond would be a great candidate for home hemodialysis, and we should speak to one of the dialysis specialists about it.

We took her advice, and honestly don't remember who it was we spoke with, but we were misinformed. In all fairness, it was a newer modality, so maybe the benefits weren't as well-known as they are today, but what I remember the most was that we would need to take 4-6 weeks of training. Meanwhile, the dialysis center Raymond was going to was looking into adding Nocturnal dialysis, which had shown great health improvements for patients, so we opted to wait for that. Inevitably, it didn't happen when a change in management at the center resulted in the decision not to move forward with that offering.

Life has a funny way of throwing us curve balls that may be frustrating at the time but are meant to disrupt and reroute us for our benefit. Our vacation to Montreal in June of 2012, was the much-needed break both Raymond and I had been looking for. Their International Jazz Festival was the draw, and the old-world charm and most delicious international foods will bring us back! As usual, when we travel, we worked with the dialysis coordinator to make arrangements for Raymond's treatments. We were staying in downtown Montreal, and there was a dialysis center close to our hotel, so we planned to utilize public transportation and walk to most of the places we wanted to go. However, that was not to be. As it turns out, because we were less than three hours driving distance to a dialysis clinic in the US, we would need to rent a car to drive to upstate NY for the two treatments Raymond would require for that vacation. The trip was wonderful, but that inconvenience flipped a switch in me.

What was that home dialysis option we had heard about? Didn't they say something about the machine being portable? Could we have taken it with us and avoided this nonsense? I started making phone calls to find the answers to my questions, and thankfully the person on the other line was able to give me so much more information that was crucial for us to know. Forget about the convenience of being able to travel with the machine; I learned that because Raymond would be able to dialyze from home five days a week, instead of three days in-center, it would be better on his heart and would give him a longer life expectancy. Well, that's all we needed to hear. They also clarified that the duration of training would depend on how quickly Raymond could pick it up, and I would need to train a fraction of the time Raymond did. Had I known the benefits earlier, I don't care if it would have been a full 4-6 weeks for me to learn, I would have made a way to make that happen.

We didn't waste any time and thankfully were able to get scheduled quickly for training for this new home modality in the summer/fall of 2012. Our training went well, and arrangements were made for a machine, chair, and supplies to be shipped to our home. The training nurse was very thorough and reassuring, and as part of the training, even came to our house for the first few sessions to make us feel even more comfortable and confident. By the 3rd treatment, Raymond felt a significant difference! He wasn't as drained after treatment, so his energy levels were much improved. It gave him more energy to work out and keep up with the kids. Knowing the benefits of home hemodialysis first-hand, Raymond later became a Patient Advocate for NX Stage to help inform other patients of this life-changing option.

2014 was my year of vision, growth, faith, courage, and change. I'll share a few highlights and save the rest of the story for another day, but 2014 set the stage for destiny to shift us in a new direction.

There were clues revealed to me throughout the year that a major shift was coming in my life. I turned 40 that April and was at the peak of my career. It was my best financial year yet. I was blessed to be able to work from home four days a week to administer Raymond's treatments, but the job I had loved was shifting in a direction that brought me more stress than joy, and I knew in my soul that the time was approaching to close that chapter to allow a new one to begin.

That summer I had the most powerful vision of my entire life. There were silhouettes of millions of people as far as the eye could see and the message was, "we've been waiting for you." That day I drew my line in the sand and set a date in the fall to submit my resignation. I shared this with Raymond, and we were in agreement, but we did not share this plan with anyone else. Then, about a month before my "jump" date, the following message came to my spirit: "You do have a choice, and you can stay at your job, but life and death are on the line." I didn't have a sense if it was Raymond's life, my life, or both, but there was no hesitation in my moving forward with my plan to resign, not fully knowing where this new journey would lead but that I needed to continue following God's breadcrumbs that were leading me.

Raymond was a model patient and was thriving, and in February 2015 we received a call from Dr. Robey letting us know that Dr. Desai nominated Raymond, and she was calling to extend tickets for us to attend the NKF AZ's DWTS gala as guests of their Nephrology practice, AKDHC. As we enjoyed the lively and energetic dance performances, I turned to Raymond and teasingly said, "Hey, that could be you dancing next year." My eyes got big, and my giggles stopped, and before I could get the words out of my mouth Raymond already knew that look on my face very well and anticipated my next words, "Wait, why not you? You can do this!" I shared this idea with Dr. Robey, who was one of the Celebrity Star dancers the year before, and her face lit up with excitement.

As you already know, Raymond did dance the following year. He was the first celebrity star dancer that was an active dialysis patient at the 10th Annual Dancing with the Stars NKF AZ Gala on February

20th, 2016…18 years to the exact day that his kidneys failed! Not only did this demonstrate the improved quality of life home dialysis can provide, and that dialysis does not have to be a death sentence, it also was an example to others that they too could beat the odds set against them.

Despite our own experiences, it wasn't until we became aware of and involved with NKF AZ through DWTS that our eyes would start to be opened to the staggering statistics surrounding Kidney Disease. Our torch of advocacy was lit, and we were inspired to start filming a documentary and create a non-profit organization to create hope and change the trajectory of kidney disease.

As I was brainstorming with my dear friend Deb about potential names for the organization, she said, "Wait, go back to that statistic you mentioned, 26 Million American's, 1 in 9 adults have Kidney Disease…that's it! 1in9." That, and meeting our incredible videographer, Taylor was how 1in9 was birthed!

You may have guessed it, but 1 in 9 American adults having Kidney Disease was one of those stats that caught us off guard. Hearing that 90% of those with CKD weren't aware was totally unacceptable to us. Diabetes is the leading cause of Kidney Disease, and high blood pressure, which is what took Raymond's kidneys, is 2nd. Kidney disease is the 9th leading cause of death in the US and kills more people than breast cancer or prostate cancer. Surprising right? It sure was to us, and we figured if this was news to us after all these years of living with it, then the general population must really be in the dark.

1in9 exists to create hope and change the trajectory of kidney disease. Our vision is to save millions of lives globally through awareness, prevention, and expedited research and development of regenerative medicine treatments and solutions.

Raymond and I are grateful for the selected co-authors who have agreed to share their "1in9" stories with you in the chapters to follow. We commend them for their courage and transparency to shine a light on kidney disease. We'll weave more of the experiences and knowledge that we have gained over the past 21 years throughout the book as well.

Over the years I've told Raymond many times that he is here for a reason. We now know why and our dance with destiny continues.

My Hero

Kenyon Scott

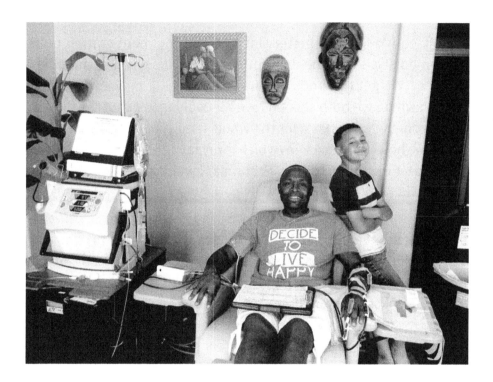

I consider myself a pretty typical teenager from a normal family. I enjoy hanging out with my friends, playing video games, teasing my little sister, going to the movies and cooking with my dad.

My first realization that our family wasn't quite as "normal" as I thought was when I was about three years old and seeing my dad in the hospital with an IV and a bunch of tubes.

In elementary school, I remember coming home and my dad having to lay down and rest after dialysis before he could get enough energy to help me with my homework, but I also remember when he was able to volunteer at my school on some of the days he didn't have to go into dialysis. Some of the kids would ask him what was wrong with his arm, which had big humps where his fistula is, and he would explain how he uses his arm to do dialysis because his kidneys don't work.

My dad feels a lot better since he and my mom started doing his hemodialysis treatments from home, and it's given us more time together. We get to bond over Marvel and Sci-Fi movies and in the kitchen where we both share a love for cooking. Most of the time we are making healthy meals for the whole family, but I've also had him teach me how to fry chicken (which is my favorite), and this year he's going to let me help make my Grandma Roveina's sweet potato pies. With enough lessons I'll eventually perfect it just like my dad has.

Over the years I've seen and learned so much that makes me even more grateful that my dad is alive. I know that because my dad is on dialysis, his immune system is weakened, so when he gets a fever, he must go to the emergency room. Many of those trips to the ER turned into hospital stays, sometimes for a few days and other times a few weeks. It can be scary, and I must be honest and admit to you that when he does go to the hospital, I prepare myself in case this is the time he dies.

Thankfully my dad continues to beat the odds as he did in 2016 when he was in the hospital for two weeks with severe sepsis and respiratory failure. My mom shielded me from seeing him while he was intubated but allowed me to visit my dad when he was recovering in the ICU after the doctors took him off the machines, and later let me see pictures so I could better understand what happened. So, whenever a new health challenge comes up, I try to remember how strong my dad is and that he's fighting to not only be there for me, my mom and my sister, but for his future grandchildren too. My dad is always telling my sister and me that when we have kids, he's going to spoil them. He jokes about how he'll load them up with candy and send them home bouncing off the walls. It always makes me smile because I can see this happening for real.

It's been exhilarating to watch my parents start and grow 1in9 and to personally be a part of it. For sure, there have been many sacrifices our family has had to make, but they've all been worth it to see how we can help others.

In 2017 our family went across the country on an RV tour. We met some amazing people and learned more than any field trip at school could ever show us! Like our visit to Dr. Ben Humphries lab at Washington University in St. Louis where we got to see kidney organoids under a microscope, and when we got to hold a prototype of the bio-artificial kidney printed with a 3D printer that Dr. Shuvo Roy and his team are creating at UCSF. I'm counting on a solution… perhaps one of these to come through and help my dad and others live a much longer life!

Whether on the road or closer to home, I've had the opportunity to meet people who have inspired me. One person that stands out is a little boy named Anthony. He was four years old when we met, and it amazed me that he had a feeding tube and had been on dialysis his whole life. Despite all the health challenges he was going through he is such a happy little boy filled with pure joy that inspires everyone he meets. I was so happy when he was able to get a kidney transplant in 2017, and I'm grateful that he's doing well.

However, I've also met and heard of people who have been scared, depressed and may think that their life is over because they are on dialysis or have learned that their kidneys are failing. I want to take a minute to encourage them.

I challenge you to find your "tribe" or at least one person that you can reach out to for guidance and support. Find at least one person who motivates you to live the best life you can. I understand it will be hard at times. You must have faith in yourself and others around you. You must make sure you are not pushing people away who are helping you not hurting you.

Instead of thinking that dialysis is a death sentence, think of it as another door being opened so you can have a second chance at life for yourself and your family. When you get scared or discouraged, think of my favorite superhero, my father, who has been on dialysis for over 20 years and doing what it takes to live his best life for me, my family, and others, including YOU!

Stay Strong

Brooklyn Scott

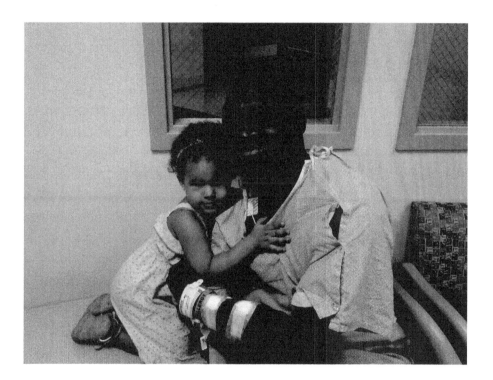

My name is Brooklyn Scott, I'm ten years old and my dad, Raymond Scott, has been on dialysis since before I was born. Some people think being on dialysis is a burden to their family, but it isn't. My dad has shown that he is a very strong person, not because of his muscles but because he builds our family up.

My mom is strong too. When my mom and dad were dating for a couple of months my dad was diagnosed with kidney failure and told her, "I have a long road ahead of me, but you don't have to be a part of it," but my mom said, "No," and is now referred to as his bulldog because she still fights for him.

Whenever my dad gets a fever, he has to go to the hospital. Most of the time I hold my emotions in, but every time he goes in, I think the worst. When he went there for a long time, it really scared me. Every time I think about sad things, I make sure my dad is okay. While I was writing my chapter for this book, I made sure my dad was okay, and he can confirm that.

My dad is on home hemodialysis. I don't clearly remember when my dad was doing in-center dialysis, but I do remember when we went to the hospital to visit him when I was one or two at the time. We have a picture from that visit, and now that he is on home hemodialysis, he looks younger than he did from back then. My dad looks amazing at age 50, and he will live a long time to come. It makes me happy when my dad talks about walking me down the aisle one day and what a fun grandpa he will be. He jokes about loading his future grandchildren with candy and sending them home bouncing off the walls, but I know better. My mom isn't going for that.

Not only does my dad feel better because he can do his dialysis at home more often than when he was going in-center, it also gives us more time together. We get to watch my favorite shows and movies together, like Black-Ish, Avatar, and Madea movies and plays - which I love because they make me laugh and always have a lesson at the end. I also get to help my mom take care of my dad while he's on dialysis by giving his readings from the machine and checking his blood pressure.

My advice to children who have a family member with kidney disease is to stay strong and know that they can live a long life. You should always encourage them to eat healthily and stay fit, and you should too. That's easy for me because I like to eat healthy food and I love to run and stay active. Sometimes I'll even join my dad when he does his work out videos in the living room, and we also have fun playing at the park.

What is a new healthy habit you and your family can adopt?

My advice to anyone with kidney disease and those on dialysis would be to live as healthy a life as you can. Know what foods to eat and which ones to avoid, stay active and stay positive. I hope my advice helps you have a better understanding of kidney disease and how to help fight this dangerous disease.

This is Brooklyn Scott signing off and thanking you for reading my chapter.

My Fight

Raymond Scott

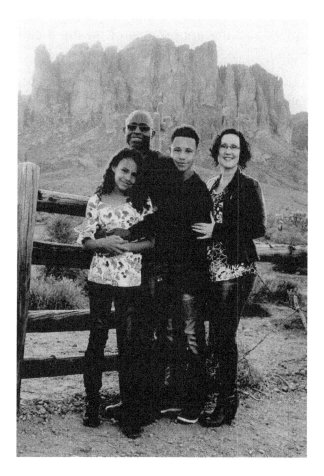

Before my kidneys failed, I did not know a thing about kidney disease. I don't think I had ever heard the word dialysis in my life. I didn't know that there were 5 stages of kidney disease until years after my kidneys failed. No one in my family, on my mother's side, was on dialysis, and I did not know anyone on my biological father's side of the family at the time that my kidneys failed. After being introduced to my biological father's family, I found out that there were several family members who had kidney disease and a couple who were dialysis patients. I was in average physical condition when my kidneys failed. I was taking my high blood pressure medications but didn't understand the importance of having a cuff to monitor regularly at home.

What I found most surprising about the main causes of kidney disease, which are diabetes and high blood pressure, is that some physicians are not making these groups of patients aware of what could happen to them if they are not addressing their blood sugar and hypertension vigilantly. Making it clear that they could end up with kidney disease, and eventually end up as dialysis patients. I also found it surprising that there were so many people of color on dialysis. It made me think of the many times as a child I heard an adult say that someone has "that sugar," or diabetes, or someone has high blood pressure. That includes my grandmother, who has been taking high blood pressure medications since I was a child. I can remember her telling me to get her medication. I even learned how to take her blood pressure manually with a BP cuff and stethoscope. For some reason, it just didn't register that I should be doing the same for me.

My immediate reaction when I learned that my kidneys had failed and I would need to begin dialysis, was "What the hell is dialysis, and how long do I have to live?" As the doctor started to explain I lost track of what he was saying and only thought of my family and how this would impact them. I then thought of my girlfriend, who is now my wife, that I met three months before kidney failure. I thought of how she was only 23 years old and had her entire life ahead of her, how unfair it would be to ask her to help me take on this disease. She picked me up from the hospital when I was released to take me home. I then told her that I was going to go back home to Charleston, SC because I knew that I had a long road ahead of me and I didn't think that it was fair for such a young woman to have to go through it with me, that she deserved better than that. She then told me, "I think that you are a great guy, I am not going anywhere." I had to give her a way out, but I was praying that she would still want to be with me. That same dedication and perseverance that she showed me, I would have to show her while dealing with this disease. The news of my kidney failure knocked me off my feet, but I was able to recover quickly with my faith, the love of an exceptional woman, and family.

My faith and my family have made the most significant difference in my longevity and quality of life as a dialysis patient. I can remember asking, "God why me?" The answer that I received was, "I have given you a wife that will be supportive, understanding, loving, devoted, and a bulldog when it comes to your care. I have given a family that will also do anything in order to support you in your care. I have surrounded you with people who love you and will pray for you at each turn, so don't ask me why ever again." I have never asked "why me" again and if my journey can help others and is what God destined as my purpose in life, then I would be willing to go back and do it all over again.

PART 2

You Are a Survivor!

Paradigm Shift

Analyn Scott

My mom is a retired nurse who spent over 20 years of her career as the nurse at a large high school in Mesa, AZ. Her office was always full because both the students and faculty knew that she believed in holistic solutions to pains that most nurses are more prone to toss a pill at. Maybe it was because she was born with one kidney and understood the adverse side effects that pain medications have on the kidneys that inspired her to combine her knowledge of trigger point therapy, massage, and a type of tiger balm to alleviate headaches, cramps, and muscle tension before resorting to a pill. Free massages? That was only one reason she was popular. She loves people and is passionate about helping others in need.

In addition to having one kidney, my mom is also a 15-year breast cancer survivor. Overall, she is healthy, not on the typical medications many other women 60+ are on, blood pressure good, blood sugar good, cholesterol good, lives a healthy lifestyle, has good health insurance, has a nursing background, and is disciplined to stay on top of her bi-annual and annual checkups with her Oncologist and PCP.

Back in 2015, I shared an opportunity for her to volunteer at one of the NKF AZ's kidney health screenings, she was eager to sign up and help. I suggested that she go ahead and sign up to get screened herself. "Oh no, I don't want to take someone's spot that needs it, someone who might not have insurance," she said. I told her that didn't matter, there were more than enough spots and it would be beneficial for her since she only has one kidney. "I'm fine," she said,

"I just went to my oncologist and PCP and I'm good." Seeing that I was still going to be persistent, she compromised and said she would bring her lab results for the Nephrologist to review. Out of curiosity, she pulled up the NKF website before the screening to see where her Glomerular Filtration Rate (GFR), which measures the level of kidney function and stage of kidney disease, would fall on the chart. To her surprise, she was at Stage 3 Kidney Disease! The GFR was clearly listed on the report, but not highlighted, and despite being a breast cancer survivor who had done chemo and radiation, and only having one kidney, neither of her physicians caught it!

During our lunch break at the kidney screening, my mom and I spoke with a few of the Nephrologists and shared her results. At first, they weren't too concerned, that it wasn't that uncommon for a woman of her age, even as she explained that she doesn't drink caffeine or alcohol, drinks plenty of water, relatively healthy...but their eyebrows rose when she said that her GFR dropped nearly 20 points from her last exam. That was a concern, and frankly, one that I would have expected her doctors to catch.

I'll never forget what one of the Nephrologists shared next. He said, "26 million American's, 1 in 9 adults have kidney disease, but 90% don't know it." WHAT? I don't remember my exact response, but I know it was one of shock, frustration, and a passionate declaration that this had to change. He continued to share, "There are 5 stages of kidney disease, stages 1-3 you can slow down or possibly reverse, but stage 4 is usually not reversible, and stage 5 is kidney failure, and dialysis or transplant is needed for survival." He then used his hand to mimic a graph that I'll try my best to give you a visual of. Picture a standard bell curve chart, or a roller coaster that from the bottom right starts it's incline up to a peak, then follows the curve into the decent down on the left side. That's what he illustrated with his hand, saying at the bottom/start, "here is stage 1, here's stage 2 (half-way to the peak), stage 3 (at the peak or top of the curve), stage 4 (half-way into decent), stage 5 (at the bottom). Do you know what happens to most people between stages 3 and 5? They die. If they make it to dialysis, they are a survivor."

Now that may not be scientific, but I'll tell you what…my mind was blown! That was one of the biggest paradigms shifts I have ever had! My mind started racing. Raymond was even more of a survivor than I thought! Raymond was part of that 90% that didn't know. How many people die of a heart attack or stroke never knowing that they had stage 3, 4, or 5 kidney disease? Raymond could have easily fallen into that group. Why am I just now learning there are 5 stages of kidney disease 17 years after Raymond's kidneys failed? How many people could have been saved if they only had a greater awareness and more could be done from a prevention standpoint? How many more people will die if a change is not made? It is time! The status quo must change!

As you continue to read the additional stories and information compiled in this book, I would be curious to learn what paradigm shifts you experienced, and/or changes you will make as a result of what you've learned.

Reflections on Kidney Disease

Marilyn Brown Coleman

My work as a school nurse was interrupted by a phone call from my daughter, Analyn. "Pray for Raymond, Mom!" was her urgent request. "He's on his way by ambulance to the hospital. His blood pressure at the urgent care was 274/190." (Raymond was Analyn's new boyfriend.) My mind was trying to wrap around those numbers. As a registered nurse, seldom did I encounter a systolic blood pressure 190 or above, yet that was the diastolic pressure—the pressure inside Raymond's heart while his heart was at rest. The upper pressure of 274 was incomprehensible! That much pressure to force the blood to flow through the blood vessels was intense. Hypertension—High Blood Pressure—the Silent Killer!!! How was this young man able to live or to survive without a major stroke or heart damage?!?!?

Reflecting on friends or patients I had known with end-stage renal disease brought images of sallow, pale faces with dry, red-rimmed eyes and extreme chronic fatigue. Quality of life and life expectancy were significantly impacted. Not the life challenges I wanted for my daughter to have to endure in a marital relationship. Raymond stated he was going to return to South Carolina and I selfishly thought, "Great! Let him go, Analyn, and find a healthy man to marry." However, I soon recognized that synergistically they face their medical challenges with courage, tenacity, and determination to live life to the fullest.

Analyn is Raymond's "bulldog," fiercely looking for healthier options for a better quality of life for him and others affected with chronic kidney disease. And, everyone loves Raymond!

What I didn't Know Did Hurt Me

Isaac Johnson

It's 1998; I'm in the prime of my collegiate football career. I'm a pre-season All-American Defensive Back at Mesa Community College. Standing 6 foot, 200 pounds I run 4.4 seconds in the forty-yard sprint. I'm on top of the world.

That's when I was introduced to a supplement called Creatine. The actual name is called Creatine Phosphate. "This supplement will get you over the hump," I was told. Of course, I gladly took it! "Who didn't want to get bigger?" I thought to myself. Well, that was a bad idea I learned about a year from that moment. At that point, I didn't know I had any issues with my kidneys.

If you've ever played a sport, then you understand that you learn mind over matter really quick. I could not physically see there was something not right with me, so it was a hard pill to swallow when I found out in 1999 that I was in stage three of Chronic Kidney Disease.

I woke up in the hospital. "What happened?" I asked the nurse. "You collapsed," she said. "I what??" I replied. I learned that the creatine I was taking for a year did not help me long term. I mean, I did gain five extra pounds. The 5 pounds was extra water weight, not muscle. Researching after the fact, I learned how bad this wonderful supplement was. Here are some of the side effects:

1. Kidney damage
2. Liver damage
3. Kidney stones

That's just the first three listed. The list goes on and on.

1999 was an eye-opening year for me. I was finishing my two years at MCC, getting ready to decide where I was going to complete my bachelor's degree and finish my college football career. Now, this? I learned there was something more important going on in life than football, especially having a two-year-old son that was counting on me (that's another story for another day). My health was at stake here. But, I was 6 ft., 205 pounds and could run a 4.4. I was being told I was "sick." "There is nothing wrong with me." I kept telling myself. I was given a lot of information that went in one ear and out the other. All I wanted to know was could I still play football, this was my ticket to paying for school. However, I realized it would also keep me away from being a father to my son, Isaac Jr. The ultimate decision was left up to me. I was faced with a tough choice, but I did what I was taught to do, to set out and finish what I started. At that time, I was in my twenties, half-way done with school and had a child to care for. Not many schools were knocking on my door, given my situation. Thankfully I was able to finish my task of getting my degree, finish my collegiate football career at New Mexico State University, and oh yeah, Isaac Jr was able to come along for that journey as well! In all honesty, I would do it again.

To me, the risk was worth the reward. I will say this, playing football at N.M.S.U was a blast. So, what I lost was 25% (more) of my kidney function during that journey. I was still big, strong and fast. Wiser to my health situation, it was time to truly give this 'illness' my undivided attention. The first step was to accept that something was wrong. The next step was to educate myself on what Chronic Kidney Disease was. That journey was long and tiring, to say the least.

Later I learned that I was born with my kidneys not functioning normally. Apparently, after I was born, I was taken from my mom for further tests. I've never learned why, or what happened, all I knew is that I've gone through life with high blood pressure. Not being educated about it, I had just figured that was my normal pressure. I learned much later in life that the high blood pressure was continually attacking my kidneys. The "silent assassin" is what I found out it was called. Very common, I learned.

Back to that accepting phase again. I had to accept that I neglected the silent assassin for the first 23 years of my life. Just as fast as I educated myself, I was on to learning how to live life with my "illness." I read books and took information classes. Needless to say, I am still on this journey of learning, coping with and living with all this.

After years of seeing a nephrologist, I was put on the transplant list in 2009. Due to insurance criteria, I had to wait until my kidney function was below 19% (I think, it was so long ago). They told me it could be up to 3 years before I would get a new kidney. No problem, "let's keep it moving along," is what I kept telling myself. I knew I could handle it. Like I said before, I looked good physically, the issue was attacking me internally. As long as I continued to monitor and take my blood pressure medication, it would be fine. Well, I finally got that call…six years later. "It's go time!" I went through the house screaming. By then I had two additional kids along the way (another story for another day). I remember calling my mom to let her know I was headed to Banner Hospital to get this kidney I had been waiting six years for.

The transplant procedure went fine. It took a couple of days for the kidney to kick in. What are a couple more days when I waited six years, right? I was up and walking around 10 hours after surgery. I'm a very competitive person and was told it would be a day or so before I could walk, which I took as a challenge. I was sent home after three days. Although my healing was ahead of schedule, it took longer to be released because the new kidney took longer to kick in. The next few months were doctor visits after doctor visits.

I felt great for about two years, that's how long the kidney lasted before I had to go on dialysis. I started with peritoneal dialysis first. That fun time consisted of being attached to a machine 14 hours a day…every day. After about a year my body decided it was time to do something different. My body was ready to get that tube removed. The least favorite choice became my last and only choice. I had to get my fistula put in so I could do hemodialysis. I had a catheter put in for temporary use while my fistula matured. Once I was able to use the fistula, I got the catheter removed. I remember standing in front of the mirror admiring all my life's battle scars, thinking how cool and strong they made me feel and look.

Fast forward to the present time. I have been on this journey since I found out back in 1999. It is now 2019; I am back on the list awaiting my second transplant…stay tuned!

This is My Story

Steve Harris

I had been hearing about high blood pressure most all my life. I had always heard something about diabetes as well. I heard but did not pay any attention to the talk. It was my father and his family from Texas who suffered from the high blood pressure, and it was my mother's family that suffered from the diabetes. So why wasn't I paying attention? I didn't feel anything, why should I be concerned. I was told that I had HBP at age 19, and later at 21, I was diagnosed with diabetes and gout. The gout was painful. I took medication for gout faithfully. But, the other stuff that came without pain, I didn't pay attention to.

In 2008, my father, at age 75, suffered kidney failure. He had a very strong heart and was placed on the kidney transplant list. Wanting desperately to help our father as best as we could, my brother and I would take dad to the dialysis center for his treatments. I did notice many people from all walks of life were being treated for kidney failure and needed to be right where they were, in a dialysis center. Still, I had not figured that I would be suffering the same fate soon.

How could I not see the writing on the wall? At 380lbs, I decided to lose weight and get serious about this kidney thing. As I reflect on my first trip to ICU, the decade that was the 80's, my days of heavy cocaine use. I believed the trip to ICU was for a cocaine overdose. I thought I would go home after a good night sleep at the hospital. I never thought about high blood pressure. I remained in the ICU for nine days while they tried every drug in the book to get my pressure under control. They could not let me leave with such high pressure.

I was used to readings of 225/105 or 195/105, 220/100. Heck, those were my normal functional numbers. But, 250/125, and it wasn't getting better. That was a real warning that I should have paid real attention to. I did, however, give up cocaine and alcohol. My life was spared because of the people in the ICU unit.

I lost 120 lbs. in an effort to save my kidneys. It was too little too late. By 2009, I had one more trip to ICU. No drugs involved. This was my third trip, and the second time I was sent straight to the hospital from a regular doctor's visit. This was the last time I would go to ICU. This time, the damage was done, and the kidney function was all but gone. My doctor prepared me for the chair that would become mine, in the dialysis center. She suggested that a fistula be prepared in my left arm for my date with dialysis. My weight loss was a good thing. Giving up the drugs and alcohol was good for me also, but it was a late effort to save my kidneys. Too late. Now I would be sitting in the center with my father.

In 2010, I was already tired of going back and forth for treatments in the center. I saw people dealing with being there in their own ways. Some watched TV, while others did puzzles. Many would try to sleep through the 3-4-hour treatment. Others would plug in their earpiece and play their music. I started to notice that everyone didn't always return on the start of the new week for treatments. People were dying. I saw others still pursuing their drinking or drug use, even up to the minute they were called for their turn on the machine. In many ways, for me, this was most depressing. I found myself asking about these people that did not show up for treatment for the past week. The answer was, he or she died in their sleep, or they had a heart attack on a Monday night because they put on too much fluid over the weekend. Taking off a lot of fluids can wreak havoc on a body. And, being in the Center for treatment was always a draining proposition. But, we had to be there. I only heard of one transplant during my time in Center

Around 2012 I was offered an opportunity to try Home Hemodialysis. What an opportunity I thought to myself. The thought of taking responsibility for my own health and treatments was just what I wanted and needed. In the Center, I had experienced this injury called infiltration (blood returned to me misses the fistula and goes directly into my muscle tissue). OUCH!!! It was the worst thing ever. I saw my arm swelling as my technician had walked off. I screamed very loud, and I was also trying to turn the machine off and keep my arm in site. It was a horrible experience. The tech was supposed to be their best in-house guy. I know he never meant to hurt me. But, the fact is, he hurt me very badly. My arm was bruised and swollen for days. I still had to go in for my treatments. In the Center was getting me down. In the Center, where the people were trying to save or extend my life as well as others, was the place that brought on depression for me. I didn't want to keep going there. People dying every month and no news ever coming about a transplant for anyone. So, when the offer came to take charge and try it at home, I jumped on that quickly.

I trained for six weeks before I was allowed to bring the NxStage System one machine home. I saw improved results the first day that I was in training on the NxStage machine. "I couldn't believe how good I was feeling." This machine brought me back into the light of hope! I did not have to stop and buy a jug of water on my way home from treatment like I had to do before. I was not drained of all my strength and fluids. They taught me to monitor and learn to read the signs that my own body would send to me. The care and attention from the North Phoenix Dialysis Center was top-notch. I mean I could feel to the core, the genuine concern that they had for me. While I hate to sound selfish, but who do we really care about? Ourselves, of course. I know that their care was for all, but what was important to me is that I was treated like I was the only concern that they had.

I lost my dad in August 2013. He had his last treatment on a Friday. He left us on that Sunday. My father had some trouble coming off the machine on that Friday. He fell, having no strength to hold himself up. I had been explaining to my father how good I felt on the NxStage machine. I was hoping we could find a way to get him on the machine, however, he was diagnosed with cancer and was taken off the transplant list. I saw all his hope vanish. He was now 80 years old and had no more desire to fight for life.

One of my mom's friend had given up hope also. She was on dialysis. For some reason, her treatments somehow involved her feet for sticking the needles. Keep in mind that a dialysis needle is like a small nail, the length of a needle but the width of a nail. The lady called her family together to announce that she was no longer going to suffer dialysis. She was dead a couple of weeks later.

2013 I lost a childhood friend who was in the Center, in his chair. He died right there in his chair. He slept and never awakened. I lost many friends and acquaintances, who were being treated in the Center by dialysis professionals, who only had their best interest at heart. Now I am at home, doing great on this NxStage machine, while all these people are dying in the Center. How the hell can I help convince people to try the Home NxStage? I offered to videotape myself doing a full 2hr treatment, and give the film to NxStage, so they can let people see how it works. More people died at my old center. In fact, most of those folks that I was in the Center with, have died. I stop counting the ones I knew at 11 or 12.

2013 had already inflicted much so hurt to my family. My youngest son had been shot and survived. My father had been taken. Now comes Thanksgiving, a time for thanks. I started feeling a bit under the weather. I had been doing everything right, so I thought. I went to a hospital to see a dying cousin. I only knew that he was an alcoholic and had been very sick lately. His feet were very swollen, like elephantiasis. He was at the Maricopa County Hospital. When I visited my cousin, there were no signs, nor did anyone say to me or anyone in my visiting party, to put on gloves, mask, and gown. My cousin was also suffering from MRSA. Due to the exposure, I went into 2014 suffering from MRSA.

My whole body and blood supply was infected with MRSA. I had Pneumonia as well. For the first time in my life, I thought I was going to die. I must have been in the hospital for about 6 weeks before they determined that I was no longer contagious and could go home. For three weeks I had to inject myself after every dialysis treatment, with more medicines to completely kill off the MRSA. I dialyzed 3-4 days a week while in the hospital. I did not quit. I did not give up. I decided then that no matter what obstacles I face, I would not quit in my quest for a lifesaving kidney. I am happy to say the least! I felt that I had beaten a super-bug even in my compromised state of health. The day came when they had to remove the injection line that lead from my neck to my heart, for that MRSA medicine. They had to remove the line in a quick, one motion attempt. All went well. So, I thought. By morning my right arm was swollen like the cartoon character Popeye! Back to the hospital. Now we must take care of a "deep vein thrombosis" blood clot.

Even though the first half of 2014 was troubling, I was still determined to get a kidney. I was concerned about my qualifications after the MRSA bout. I started asking about how long must one wait for a kidney; how long can I live on this great machine? I started working out again. I wanted to keep my numbers looking good. I wanted to keep looking and feeling good. I started writing again. I wrote songs and outlines to stories that I will want to finish up in time. Anything to stay busy. I started preparing taxes again, this time for pay.

December 29th 2014, I awoke around 2 a.m. to the smell of smoke. I got up and felt my way to my lights. I turned them on, but the smoke was so thick that I could not see in front of me. I manage to call 911 and was instructed to get myself and anyone I can out of the house immediately. I awaken my 6'8" 360lb. baby boy, got my NxStage, and exited the house as the firemen were coming thru with axes and hoses. The house was lost. On January 1st, 2015, New Year's Day, I was moving into a hotel for a long stay while my house is being rebuilt. I had my son and my NxStage Machine. To me, that was all that mattered.

2015, my life is again in turmoil. I am living in a hotel that is not kind to me regarding my NxStage Machine. Of course, I felt something different coming at me. Felt like a little bit of racist behavior going on, but I don't want to call it out. Maybe I was simply feeling a little sensitive. They wanted me to find somewhere else other than their hotel to dump my used supplies. But guess what, I am not going anywhere. If we must be defiant with anyone, then let's get it on. I was tired, I was deflated, but I was anything but beaten. So, I fought with the management, my insurance company, and anyone else who wanted to deny me a hotel room because I had my machine and supplies. They also had to receive my deliveries of supplies and bring them to my room. I had seen what depression could do, and I would refuse anti-depression meds. My uplift must come from my desire to keep going. I did get sick while in the hotel. Once I could move back into my new home, things began to change a little bit.

In 2016, things started to look better. Calls from Mayo Clinic began to come in. They were giving me stats and telling me about deciding on a kidney. They informed me that I might be close to receiving one. I remember getting my first call and offer of a kidney. I was so excited. They talked to me about the condition of the kidney. It wasn't the best kidney, but it was a working kidney. That's what I was thinking. I was about to say yes to the kidney but decided to wait a moment and review what I was taught about the different scores on kidneys. This kidney was not a high-scoring kidney. My doctor declined the kidney. He explained to me that since I had been doing so well on treatments, that I could wait for a better one to come along. I agreed because Mayo had been right on everything thus far. Two or three more offers would come, and again my doctor would turn them down.

In December of 2016, I found my co-pilot, Nikesha. A young lady that I had known for years. She is a writer also. I liked that a lot. Although I had known her for several years as a Poker player, I had not known that she was also a person who loved writing. We had enjoyed each other's company for some time in a casual way, never intimately. I had considered myself useless, inadequate and not fit for any type of serious relationship. Thank God someone else had more sense that I did. Regardless of my health, wealth, notoriety or anything else, the young lady wanted me in her life. I can only thank God, for bringing me a worthy companion. That was December of 2016.

In January 2017, I got news that a screenplay that I wrote in 2003 was being reviewed at the 2017 Hollywood Black Film Festival. Imagine that! A script my partner Chris and I had written 14 years earlier while working together at the Dept. of Revenue, was finally getting noticed. It was an amazing experience, to say the least. Walking the red carpet in Hollywood with known stars was a dream that happened. My NxStage was there right with me. Thousands of contestants involved with movie making in one way or another were there, meeting, greeting, and networking. An actor and producer showed up at the festival to inquire about our screenplay. Our script was the talk of the festival. We signed an option agreement giving this actor permission to attempt to get this script into production.

July 2017, Mayo Clinic called again about a kidney. This time I wasn't too excited. I had been thru this before. I had the bags packed. We took the ride all the way to Mayo clinic again. This time I got to meet the doctor, the guy who had been turning down kidneys. He said to me, "This is the one, Mr. Harris." He looked like a football running back for a college team. He was young, Black, and looked to be in great shape himself. There is nothing like the feeling of relief. That's the feeling I had the moment he said, "I got you, Mr. Harris," and all fears and anxiety were relieved. I was ready. At last the operation would happen.

At this moment in time, I was experiencing an enormous amount of joy, and I just wanted to thank God over and over all evening. I was giving thanks and praying as they were telling me to count backward.

I have told you that I never really experienced much pain as I went through these years of failed kidneys. Well now that the kidney operation was a success, and Big Steve is going to be all right, LET THERE BE PAIN! During the four months of recovery, I had pain most of the time. I will not disclose the pain of recovery, because I would not want anyone to be discouraged about the process. I must say if I had to go thru the operation again, I would surely do so.

My message is clear.

The warning signs must be taken seriously, and a person must act on those signs even if there is no pain associated with the signs. HOPE is a huge factor. Staying hopeful and refusing to become depressed was key, and a big factor in the success I've experienced. Hope along with prayer defeated any depression that tried to creep in on me.

Now, I am well, my numbers are good. I have a new career at 62, a new love in my life, and opportunities are all around me. NEVER GIVE UP ON YOUR LIFE!

To date, we are still in the process of getting this movie made. I have new hopes in new areas of my life. I never gave up, and I am still here.

The Prayer Jar

Shellisa Multrie

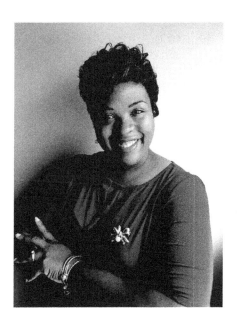

"Your kidney function is declining," said a young and very upbeat nephrologist at a routine check-up. We were newly married, after only dating for about six months. Nothing was wrong. Tim did not feel sick. It was just a part of his life after receiving a kidney transplant back in 2001. He had to do periodic blood work, and they would make adjustments when needed. He was 36 years old now, a divorced dad of two, now newly married, new to Charlotte, NC and a new superintendent at his company. For now, there was nothing to panic about, only something to watch.

I remember being a little concerned because I already knew what dialysis was like. My mother ironically had been on dialysis for about seven years, due to a complication with Lupus, but she no longer needed it. My mind wondered about what was ahead. I did not fully understand that there was a possibility that a kidney could stop working after transplant. The amount of learning that would follow would be tremendous and unclear. What we knew for sure was that at some point the decline in kidney function would one day lead to returning to dialysis. How long would it be? We had no idea, but for now, we would settle into our new life as husband and wife with a blended family.

We both came with small families. Tim had two daughters, and a bonus girl from his first marriage. My son from a previous relationship was also a part of the bunch. About eight years separated Tim and me in age, but that did not seem to matter much at the time. Our new life was nothing out of the ordinary. We both had thriving careers, managed our home life and enjoyed many new adventures together. After having decided not to grow our family any further, we found out that we were expecting. We thought this was God's way of laughing at our plans and giving us what He thought we needed despite our efforts to "medically plan" our way out of more children. Savannah Grace would be born almost a year and a half after we said, "I do." She was perfectly healthy, noisy, wide-awake, tiny, and all the things that new babies are supposed to be. Indeed, she was a gift to us, and our family expanded with just enough love for her. Tim called her pumpkin (he still does), and often would marvel at her little features that reminded him of his mother and his other two daughters.

After a Thanksgiving visit to my hometown, we were about to enjoy Sunday dinner when Tim noticed that he had a tingle in his left arm. It would not stop, and I grew very concerned. We packed up our five-year-old Jay, and two-month-old Savannah and headed to the hospital. Our twelve-year-old was still with her mother from her holiday visit. After what seemed like forever, we learned that Tim was experiencing a heart attack. It was unfathomable to me. He was not even 38 yet.

We had a brand-new baby, had been house hunting to accommodate our larger family, and we had just gotten back from vacation, for goodness sake. It all became a blur for us as they scrambled to find out just what had happened. I do remember that one of the tests that they performed posed some risk to his kidney because of the dye used in the procedure. The team would discover that Tim had a heart attack on a minor branch artery on the bottom of his heart. They would recommend treating with medicine only. When we returned home, we would quickly realize that the terms "major and minor," when thinking through recovery from a heart attack meant nothing. It was all serious. It was evident that it had taken a toll on Tim. Going up the stairs was a challenge at first, and he tired quickly. He would recover over the next several weeks, and we would adjust to our new normal, with a new diet and exercise.

By the summer of 2008, we were planning to begin the process to start peritoneal dialysis, which uses the peritoneum, a cavity in the abdomen to deposit and remove a sugary fluid that cleans waste from the body. It required surgery to insert a tube into the abdomen, a machine to warm and measure input/output, as well as an endless supply of fluid. The fluid came in three strengths and required three large bags for each treatment. The fluid was delivered monthly and usually amounted to about 30-40 boxes. Our first delivery came in late September that year just after Savannah's first birthday. The delivery was quite daunting. There were boxes, medical equipment, and so many other things delivered to our home. We had been scared straight in our training classes about the need for sterilization and the dangers of infection. It seems like our life was taking yet another turn and we had absolutely no control of what was happening. Our only choice was to adhere to changes to keep Tim alive and well while we waited on a new kidney.

By now, we were making friends with our local hospital's transplant team. We were approved for a kidney transplant. I still remember getting a letter from my employer at the time, sharing our insurance would cover our transplant expenses. They told us that it would take 2-3 years based on Charlotte's waitlist. That may seem like a long time but, it's important to note that this was Tim's second transplant which meant that he had even more antibodies to consider than a first timer. This would make him a more difficult match. Our best chance would be for a living donor. A living donor kidney can last 25 years or more while a deceased donor kidney may be limited to seven to ten years. His first kidney had lasted about seven years so I made the decision that we would need to find a living donor to give us more time and decrease our risk for rejection. The team provided donor packets for us and some general guidelines for people who would like to try to donate a kidney to Tim. Immediately I figured that we just needed to find a donor, and with all of Tim's siblings and family, plus our own network of friends that this would be a piece of cake…right?

We had friends, and a few family members try to donate unsuccessfully over the years. They were from all over the country, and for that, we will always be grateful. We quickly realized that most people do not understand how kidneys work, that you only need one to survive and that a life lived indefinitely on dialysis was not desirable. We found ourselves trying to educate people on kidney disease. The more we learned, the more we shared with others. There were so many things to remember and understand while living on dialysis. We made sure to continue to travel when we could and make the best of things. At this time, Tim was working full time and attending college online, which was amazing to his medical team. Each day, he would work 12-14 hours a day followed by nine hours of dialysis overnight. He would eat dinner, take a shower and hook up to his dialysis machine. He would then complete homework, help kids with homework and get rest before starting the entire routine over the next day. It was grueling, but Tim has always been a man committed to taking care of his family and going to work. He was not going to let something like kidney failure stop him.

We would do peritoneal dialysis for four years. In the summer of 2012, Tim got sick. His peritoneum was no longer cleaning properly. He would need to transition hemodialysis as soon as possible. By now, we had buried his mother who died suddenly in December 2010; Tim had graduated from a business program and was working a less stressful job that he loved. I was laid off from my job in the fall of 2011 and trying to find a new normal. It was quite possibly the worst possible time ever. We decided that Tim would need to stop working and we would instead focus on getting him healthy. We spent that summer of 2012 trying to qualify for disability and adjusting to in center dialysis three days a week. At this point, I felt helpless, and if I felt that way, I am sure that Tim was feeling even worse. We were without health insurance other than Medicare for Tim and Medicaid for the kids. When you need a kidney transplant, you must carry two forms of insurance, no exceptions. This is largely because of the cost of the medicines that you will need to be on for the rest of your life as well as the procedure and other medical care needed. In essence, the hospital made us inactive on the list for 2.5 years while I looked for full-time work.

We do not talk much about the struggles that we went through during this time, but we had to trust God because nothing on paper looked promising. How we made, it was a miracle. We tried to focus on keeping Tim healthy enough to be active again whenever I was able to go back to work full time. There are moments when the pressure was so great, so intense that I do not have words. We lost so much during this time, and we would lose more over the next year. We opened a small business, and it just bled money. We needed every dime, and we prayed for more. We worked so hard to make the ends not meet, but instead, we were only able to get the ends close enough to each other so that we could feel some sense of normalcy. Doctor visits were routine during this time. Being inactive on the transplant list did not leave the doctors with much to do for us. We had been on dialysis for over six years before I went back to work full time at the end of 2014. While on my final interview, I honestly could not muster up any energy to negotiate on my salary. My only non-negotiable was health insurance, and I was so happy to receive it that I didn't care what they paid me. I just wanted to get us back on the active transplant list. We went active again in 2015.

By this time, I am sure that our transplant team was not feeling very hopeful for a match for us. They did not seem to have enthusiasm or spark for our case. We continued to have hope. I am not sure of what Tim prayed for during this time, but I did not pray for a kidney every day. I did not have to. I had expressed my desires to God early on, and I believed that God would do it, somehow. Occasionally I would write it on a prayer card, grocery store pin-up, wishing well note, whatever. I would mention it if a group I was a part of was soliciting prayer requests. It just did not consume me because I just trusted that He would do it.

My belief was not without bouts of sadness and despair. Whenever Tim would be hospitalized (and there would be many, many times), I would grow tense. The amount of coordination when he went to the hospital would overwhelm me. What time was it? Can we wait to go to the emergency room until the kids go to sleep? Should I take them to my cousins now? How long will we have to stay? How much should I pack for everyone while we are away? Who can keep the dog? How much money do we have? There was a lot of stress, and often Tim would feel like I resented him getting sick. In reality, my concerns about all of this "stuff" just helped me not focus on the seriousness of his illness. Every time he got sick, somewhere in my heart I wondered, "How much longer God? I don't think we can keep this up too much longer."

Life got better in many ways after I went back to work, but Tim continued to grow sicker. Dialysis is not a long-term strategy for survival. The human body begins to have other challenges after being on dialysis for long periods. Sometimes your dialysis access fails, you develop other conditions like pulmonary hypertension, gastroparesis, achy joints, rashes, poor circulation, just all kinds of things. We were just doing our best to deal with everything that came our way. Our kids were getting older and living with dialysis was just a part of our lives. They knew the hospital drill by now, and they did not ask me many questions when I returned home alone without dad. We just tried to keep going. That is all that we could do. Still, in the quiet moments when I would find myself alone in my thoughts, I wondered, "How much longer God? He isn't getting any better."

In April 2017, we received a call that there might be a possible match for us. I do not remember much of what they said but I know we called everyone we knew, made the ceremonial Facebook post and got to the hospital as soon as possible. For nearly 24 hours, we waited while they poked and prodded Tim, hooking him up to an excruciating machine responsible for measuring his heart pressures. He was so uncomfortable, but he fought through it because that in comparison to what we had been going through was nothing. The kidney was late getting to the hospital due to a flight delay…odd, I know. When it arrived, they ran a final test to see if all the computer matches were accurate. It turns out there was one marker that did not produce the results that the surgeon was looking for and just like that, our hopes were dashed. We were devastated. No kidney. You can go home now. We left the hospital with a Tim in physical pain and our hearts broken. The worst part I still feel was telling our babies that there was no kidney for us. They were so excited when we left to go to the hospital and now, we would have to break their hearts too with the news.

I wish that was the end of it because surely that would have been enough. Shortly after we did not get the kidney, we had a follow-up appointment with our nephrologist. He explained that based on Tim's heart function, he feared that he would not survive the surgery if another kidney ever became available. The transplant team decided to take us out of contention due to Tim's pulmonary hypertension. Our emotions could not be contained, and we both began to cry uncontrollably. This just did not seem fair or make any sense. We had waited for almost nine years already, and now, we were no longer being considered? We had insurance. I was working again; we had followed everything that they said for us to do. It was as if we had been disqualified from a race that we had been training for before we even suited up. We did not even get to walk on the field. This pain was worse than what we had experienced at the hospital. It felt final and cold. I quietly wondered in a secret, quiet corner of my mind, "God, why are you letting this happen? How will we get a kidney now?"

The transplant office encouraged us to seek out other more advanced hospitals that might possibly consider and list us. They recommended Johns Hopkins and Duke University Hospital. In the summer of 2017, we would travel to both for evaluation. Both offered us hope, but they also presented a new challenge. If we were to receive a kidney from either, we would have to get to them and be able to stay indefinitely. Johns Hopkins was a six-hour drive for us, but luckily, my uncle lived an hour away and was open to us staying with him if needed. Duke was a little over two hours away. At this point, we did not care because we needed to live. We were willing to do whatever it took. We heard from Duke first. They were very optimistic about Tim's heart condition and his viability for transplant. Every person there was seemingly unbothered by our condition. Johns Hopkins was also very positive but needed additional tests completed before they made their decision. We were listed at Duke University Hospital in October 2017 for a kidney transplant.

This new hope was just what we needed to keep us moving forward. By the end of 2017, we decided that we would live while on dialysis. We would no longer "wait" for a kidney to do the things that we wanted to do. Instead, we would just move forward, and whenever it came, we would be ready. We booked a family trip for the first time in many years. We started making plans to move out of our rental house and buy a home again. We focused more on our faith. Tim even started working a part-time job. We ended 2017 with hope for a future. Tim found a home for us, and we started the process of building. We were working hard to pay off bills and take back our lives. We followed our renal diet strictly and managed through gastroparesis. The months were flying by, but we had hope, and that was enough.

In June 2018, Tim was not feeling the best. In fact, he seems to be growing weak suddenly. We had seen similar times before and it was normally because he had too much fluid on him. This is a common issue and guessing game for dialysis patients. Too little fluid can cause cramping, too much can cause shortness of breath, fatigue and other issues. This time was a little different because he did not show many signs of fluid overload, but he was not doing well either. One Friday night, a friend was coming over to bring some things by for our daughter, so Tim went to go lay down.

I was chatting with her when I heard Tim saying something. I could not make out what it was, but he seemed to be yelling but nothing that made sense. Something just did not seem right, so I came up to check on him, and he was covered in sweat and sliding off the bed. He fell back and seemed to be losing consciousness. I screamed for my friend Denise to come and help me and for my son to call 9-1-1. We were able to get Tim on the floor, but he could not help us at all. His eyes kept opening and closing, he was soaked in sweat, and I had never seen him this way. "Don't leave me," I kept repeating. "I love you." We were always able to get to the hospital on our own, but now, I needed help getting him to the floor. He started to cry and so did I. For the first time in all our years together, I was scared that he was leaving me, and I could not do a single thing about it.

When the paramedics arrived, they started working on him, gave him oxygen and got him to the ambulance. Our support system came and handled the kids and Denise brought my car to the hospital so that I could ride in the ambulance. The entire ride I was nervous. I did not know what was happening or what had gone wrong. I did not have time to prepare. He was scared, and so was I. We were completely lost. When we arrived at the hospital, they had gotten him stabilized. He was asking about the kids and if they were okay. He was worried about how we were doing. The doctor we had that evening, Dr. Belazairre, was one of the most compassionate that we had experienced over the years. She read our medical history like it was a story or a complex puzzle that unfolded to what she saw before her. They attributed Tim's symptoms to fluid overload. They treated and released him the next day. He missed the kids leaving for their summer trip that day. They traveled together for the first time, and as much as I was going to miss them, I was more emotional about them leaving before Tim could come home from the hospital. He was released on Saturday, June 28, 2018, to return home. You must understand that this time was so much scarier than any other visit to the hospital. I could not ask God when or how…I was too scared. I was never afraid of losing Tim until now. I tried to push those fears aside and ask God to make a way.

We went to church that Sunday and then to lunch. He felt so much better, it was amazing. The next few days were normal. He went to work, and so did I. We were determined to enjoy this time together while the children were away. The morning of the Independence Day came, and we were determined to live a day free from it all. Free from disease, work, worry…everything. We went to the gym together, furniture window-shopping and for a free smoothie at Clean Juice. We had never been to Clean Juice but decided to check out the free treats. Once we arrived, we learned that they were out of free smoothies, but we ordered some anyway. We noticed a prayer jar on the counter, and as always, I filled out a prayer request and wrote, "Tim Needs a Kidney." This was normal for me. We left and cooked out at home, just the two of us. I was making all kinds of cooking videos while Tim was on the grill. After dinner, he laid out for a nap. His phone rang twice and the house phone too. The third time the phone rang I nudged him to answer and to our surprise it was Duke's transplant office calling. "We think we have a match for you…," they said.

They asked us a battery of questions about Tim's current health and any issues that were going on. They told us to sit tight and wait for them to call us back with further instructions. This time we made just a few calls to share with family and a handful of friends that we had received the call. The next 48 hours were slow and just a series of manufactured distractions to help us not focus on the phone ringing. We visited every furniture store in the city, packed, and cleaned our home, just anything to keep us distracted.

On Friday, July 6 at around 5 pm, Duke called and told us to make our way to the hospital. We put our bags in the car and hit the road. We arrived a few hours later and were admitted to the hospital. The entire time we were expecting to wait again and undergo tests like the ones we had endured in April 2017. They did bloodwork and moved us to a different floor. The room on the transplant surgery floor was bare. It was quiet. It was late. We waited and waited, but everyone seemed calm. We were wondering when they would hook him up to the painful machine in his neck again to monitor his heart pressures, but they did not.

Finally, an anesthesiologist came to talk with us about what to expect, and while I remember him being rather funny and very easy going, I only remember feeling like, "Is this really happening this time?" I did not want to get excited because I knew the disappointment from the last time. The nurses rattled a bunch of numbers to the surgeon when he arrived. He apologized just like the anesthesiologist about the long wait. After just a few more minutes, they wheeled Tim away for his kidney transplant. I went to rest in the waiting room for what would be about five hours. Somehow, in my mind, I thought they would come back and share that they could not do the surgery. After some time, I drifted off to sleep on a tiny little couch in a nearly empty room with a television playing in the background.

Dr. Bradley Collins woke me early Saturday, July 7 to share that the transplant had been successful. He explained in the most compassionate way about how the procedure went and how he worked within the way God made Tim's body. It was at that time that I realized that Tim had been given new life in the way of a kidney on his mother's birthday. This was the confirmation that I needed that this was for real. After almost ten years of waiting, God had answered our prayers. Our lives are forever changed, and we are grateful to our donor family who allowed their loved one to extend Tim's life.

This adventure has been wild and unscripted, painful but purposeful. We are a living testimony of God's faithfulness through it all. Though kidney disease has been a part of our entire marriage, we are hopeful for a bright future and a chance at life. Grateful is simply not enough to explain how we feel, but it is a start.

PART 3:

Out of the Shadows

"The Funky Diabetic"

Analyn Scott

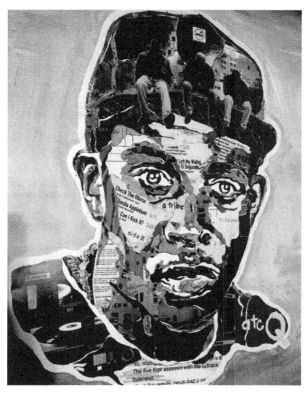

"Funky Diabetic"
by Kris Rhymes - KRhymes Artistry

"When was the last time you heard a funky diabetic?" If you're a 90's Hip Hop fan like I am then, you'll likely think immediately of A Tribe Called Quest and hear Phife Dawg's voice in your head rapping that lyric. Maybe he didn't give much thought of it at the time when he wrote the lyrics, but he deserves major props for speaking out. He bravely did so a few times over the years as his battle with diabetes progressed, and like so many other diabetics, it led to kidney disease, kidney failure, and ultimately to his death on March 22, 2016, at the age of 45.

Phife's given name was Malik Taylor, and I was saddened when I heard the news of his passing. Reading the articles published after his death I learned that the kidney his wife had donated to him in 2008 had failed in 2012 and he had been back on dialysis three days a week. I couldn't help but wonder if he was ever informed about the benefits of dialyzing more frequently and given the option of home dialysis. My heart went out to his widow, Deisha. I didn't know her personally but knew she gave much more than just a kidney to him during their journey together.

The link between diabetes and kidney disease is not recognized by most people, even though it's the leading cause of kidney disease. It may also surprise you to know that diabetes accounts for nearly 44% of patients newly diagnosed with kidney failure and that 35% of adult diabetics 20 years or older have Kidney Disease. If these statistics shock and alarm you, they should. As we continue to see diabetes on the rise, you guessed it; we see an increase in those with Kidney Disease.

March is Kidney Disease Awareness month, and 1in9 hit the road in 2016 for an RV tour across the East Coast, which included a stop in New York City to pay tribute to Phife Dawg on the one-year anniversary of his passing.

Artist Kris Rhymes of KRhymes Artistry, in collaboration with 1in9, showcased the "Funky Diabetic," a piece from his new "Cover to Cover" Collection at the tribute event.

"I want to bring support to 1in9 through my art, and pay tribute to Phife Dawg, not just because A Tribe Called Quest is my favorite

Rap group, but to shine a light of awareness on Kidney Disease and diabetes." - Kris Rhymes

If you have diabetes, are pre-diabetic, have a family history of diabetes, high blood pressure or kidney disease. I recommend that you ask your doctor to run two simple tests to get a baseline on your kidneys. A blood test to check your GFR and a urine test called ACR or "albumin-to-creatinine ratio." You are your best advocate, so be proactive and request these be monitored, compared and the status explained to you at your annual physicals.

Inspiring a Legacy of Change

Micaiah & Micah Thomas

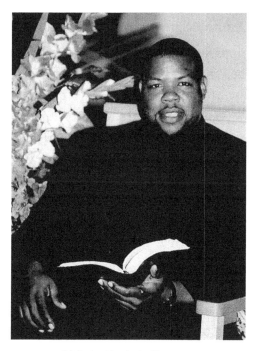

Bishop Alexis A. Thomas

Beyond the Headlines

January 18, 2018, our world was rocked, and our lives forever changed. The impact was felt across Phoenix, the State of Arizona and across the nation the next day and for weeks to follow as the headline "Bishop Alexis Thomas of Pilgrim Rest Baptist Church dies at 50", and others like it began to circulate across local and national media.

An excerpt from the church's press release proclaimed: "Pilgrim Rest Baptist Church is saddened to announce the death of Bishop

Alexis A. Thomas, a distinguished member of the clergy, Pastor, husband, and father, who passed away on January 18, 2018, at the young age of 50. Bishop Thomas, a child prodigy who preached his first sermon at the age of 7, transformed Pilgrim Rest Baptist Church, located at 1401 E Jefferson Street in Phoenix, Arizona, from a small congregation of 200 to one of the most prominent African-American ministries in the Southwest with over 4,000 members.

Bishop Thomas was a dynamic preacher and a passionate orator. He received his license to preach the gospel at the tender age of 7. After serving as an Associate Minister at the Pilgrim Rest Baptist Church, he was named Senior Pastor in 1984 at the age of 16, a historic event in the State of Arizona. Bishop Thomas held a Bachelor of Science Degree in Biblical Studies from Southwestern Bible College in Phoenix, Arizona. Bishop Thomas authored and published his book titled "A Child Shall Lead Them" in 2005. His book chronicled the journey God had led him through in the first 36 years of his life and left the reader waiting to read the rest of his journey."

He was all these things and so much more to us; he was our Dad! We are twins and the youngest of his five sons from his first marriage to our mother, Doretta Thomas. We have come together to share our collective story and continue dad's legacy of service by sharing part of his journey that wasn't in the headlines. Just as his life was, our father's death will be a light for others!

The Two Calls

Our mother had been trying to call our dad all day because he was supposed to meet her for a consultation. The day before, our mother had been diagnosed with Stage 1 cancer and after our mom and dad talked about it earlier that Wednesday morning, he told her to round up all the boys, and they would tell us together. So, the last time we all spoke to our father was that Wednesday evening at 6:30 pm.

That was the first call, which none of us handled too well. We pretended to, but after hanging up the phone call with our parents, I cried and couldn't stop thinking of the possibility of losing our mother, the woman who opposite of our dad, had always been the healthiest person we knew, a vegan and an avid health nut. However, dad assured us all that he would be there to support our mother every step of her journey. However, as God would have it, dad was called to his eternal home early Thursday morning!

The second call came Thursday when our mother called crying hysterically, telling me to find my twin and meet her out at dad's house. I calmly asked her to slow down and tell me what was wrong, she didn't want to tell me dad had passed, but I told her to tell me so that I could get my brother. I already knew what happened; I just needed her to say it. After she told me, I went to get my brother, and we met everyone out at dads.

I remember walking in, all these people I didn't know just standing around and then I saw my mother in the living room on the floor crying and looking lost. I asked to see him but was told we had to wait for the coroner to pronounce his death. I remember walking outside to the back yard in disbelief but also relief; our dad would no longer be sick, no longer be up for days at a time and no longer have a dresser filled with medicine bottles. I remember when we were allowed to go back in to see him, the position he was lying in. I remember thinking that dad was known and loved by thousands of people, but he died alone in a little room all by himself. That was hard to take. He did so much for so many, and he died alone!

The Downward Spiral

Watching our father's health spiral down from the time we were kids was difficult. We were probably 10 or 12 years old when we first noticed there were health issues, but as we got into our teenage years, from around 16 and up, we knew things were getting worse. Then at 21, dad was gone.

When we were younger and tried to bring our concerns to his attention, he would say we didn't know what we were talking about, but as we began to mature, he could no longer hide some things from us. Many times, he would tell us he was getting things under control or that we were over-exaggerating. We saw him wither away right before our eyes.

There wasn't just one illness or one cause, it was diabetes, not eating properly, the diet sodas exercising off and on. Then the high blood pressure, heart problems, and kidney disease. However, he never really addressed any of it. We would see all the medication in his bathroom, from pain pills for his neuropathy to all kinds of medicine and the insulin in the refrigerator. We could see his health getting worse, why couldn't he? A couple of summers we stayed with our dad because he lived closer to our jobs. This would be an eye-opening experience for more than one reason. We would see him not sleep for three or four days at a time, staying up all night singing and beating on the walls or tables like they were drums. When he didn't sleep, we couldn't either! We suspected that some of the medications prescribed to him were probably keeping him up where others were trying to bring him down, so at times he was put into a state of euphoria. It was so sad to see him like that because this was our dad who we thought was the strongest man in the world.

Dad missed so many events that we were having because he just couldn't cope out in public, and often when he would come, he would have to leave early because he wasn't feeling good. There were times we would go out with him, and he would become ill and unable to drive, so we would have to drive him home and put him in bed. We were all so afraid he would become ill while driving and hurt himself in an accident, or worse, hurt someone else.

Our emotions were all over the place; we would get so angry at him at times because he wouldn't take better care of himself and he would keep us up all night. Then we would look at him with sadness, sometimes having to shut ourselves away and cry because he seemed unable to help himself, almost like a baby. There would be times when we would have to laugh again so we did not cry.

We would take him to lunch and tell him that he had to get help, or we didn't want to be around him to see him hurt himself or someone else, but nothing worked for long. He would eventually go back to not taking his medicine or taking too much, and be right back at his childlike state, where we would again hold his hand and try our best to take care of him. So much of our youth was taken away from us because of his sickness and before becoming adults we found ourselves being the parent at times taking care of our ailing grown child.

We would call our mom, and she would try to talk to him. He would listen for a little while, and at one point almost agreed to go away to a holistic health center to address his health issues and learn how to make the necessary lifestyle changes to improve his health, but ultimately would decide not to. We believe that so much of him not wanting to go away and get help was this perception that he had to appear to be this perfect man of God in front of the people, while on the inside he was dying right before our eyes. If only he knew that it wasn't too late to ask for help and people would gladly be there for him like he was for them. That they would love him just the same, how so many of them would be able to relate and be empowered because they were fighting similar battles, and how perhaps additional solutions could have been brought to his attention.

This didn't all happen overnight. Dad had diabetes as a teenager, and I don't think it was addressed until he and our mom got married, so we don't know how long he went without proper health care and medication to help keep it under control. As the years went by, he started having trouble with high blood pressure, but he continued to constantly eat fried foods, fatty foods, diet sodas, sweets, everything that he wasn't supposed to eat. High cholesterol was next, followed by heart problems. Since he never took control of the diabetes, he started having diabetic neuropathy in his feet, which is common in people who have had diabetes awhile. I think that's when all the mixing of the medicine came into play, he had the medicine for the neuropathy and the pain medication, and they started getting him incoherent. He would forget how much and which medicine he took and would go on days without resting or sleeping.

Dad was told a few years ago that he had kidney disease and that his kidneys were only functioning at 20%, but he kept on trying to tell us everything was okay. Even that wasn't enough of a wakeup call to make some necessary changes. He didn't cook and didn't have anyone that cooked for him unless he would hire a chef for a couple of weeks and then go back to the bad eating habits.

We loved our dad so much and would do anything for him, he was a loving father that took care of us, our family and what seemed like the whole world, but just couldn't take care of himself. We remember our mother asking him if he wanted to live and he said to her in a very sheepish way, "I guess so." So, I think at some point our dad decided he was ok with dying without trying to live. He will miss our college graduations, his chance to perform our marriages, to see more of his grandchildren born. We feel so robbed of our time with him because at 50, that's when he should've been getting a new lease on life and sharing his wisdom with all of his sons, not dying and leaving us to figure out things on our own. There are some things that only our dad could do for us.

Illuminating the Path to Change

One thing our father tried to hide from the public is just how sick he was, but those who were really close to him knew. He had such a powerful ministry, and to see his mission cut short has been totally devastating. Had dad been more open and taken better care of his health, we believe he would have had another decade or more. His death taught us that when we don't take charge of our health, we are at risk to prematurely abort our assignment. People may say if God wanted it to be, he could have done something, but God gives us all free will.

Dad had known he was not in good health, so he started talking to all his sons about what to do when something happened to him. He told two of us about the financial piece, and that mom was over that, and then he told Micah, "be a better man than I was."

Since dad's passing, we are constantly having random folks come up and tell us how he helped them when they first moved to Phoenix, how he prayed for one of their family members, how he would reach in his pocket and give someone money after talking to them. He married, buried, counseled, taught, and preached to millions, but unfortunately couldn't be transparent enough to say I'm in trouble. So, we're without our dad at a time we are becoming men and need his guidance the most. And, we are left wondering, had our dad confronted his health head-on and turned some things around, how many more lives could he have influenced, empowered and changed?

We miss dad terribly and believe it is our right and our duty to share with others how important it is to take care of their health. If by shining a light on what he went through can help someone else, it would put a silver lining of purpose around some of these painful memories. We hope that we can help raise awareness for diabetes and kidney disease and empower others to come out of the shadows knowing they're not alone. We believe it's important for the public to know that diabetes has a domino effect triggering other issues and diseases throughout the body, including, and far too often, kidney disease.

Through this experience, my brothers and I have decided that our generational health issues died that night with dad. We will not die early because we neglected our health. We will not only take control of our health, but we will also continue to shine our light and lend our voices to help others!

Too many of our relatives have been taken before their children turned 25. Therefore, we have declared that the diseases that took our father, our uncle and that our grandfather is currently dealing with will stop there. Our generation, that of our children and beyond will take a stand to change the health history of our family. Because of the awareness we now have, my brothers and I vow to take better care of our health so that we can live to see our children well beyond their 25th birthdays!

The last of Bishop Alexis Thomas & Doretta Thomas' five sons. Currently attending Arizona State University majoring in Political

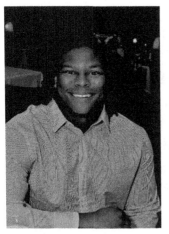

Science, I'm an active member of Delta Tau Delta Fraternity. Former member of the Chandler-Gilbert Community College Model United Nations Team where I had the opportunity to speak at the 2017 Model United Nations of the Far West Opening Plenary Session in San Francisco representing my school. I started working as a lifeguard for the City of Phoenix in 2012 then moved to diving coach and last as an assistant manager. Upon graduation my desire is to work for the United Nations. One of my goals in life is to shed light on the importance of taking care of your physical health which untimely took my father and my plan is to end that unhealthy cycle.

Micaiah Emil Thomas

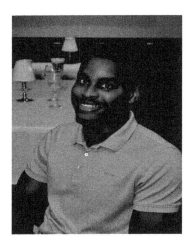

I am the fourth son of Bishop Alexis Thomas and Doretta Thomas. I'm a senior at Grand Canyon University majoring in Finance and Economics graduating fall of 2019. I'm looking forward to pursuing a career in Investment Banking upon graduation. As a high school senior at Estrella Foothills High School I held the record for the best times in five swimming events. I was also one of the youngest lifeguards and swim coaches for the City of Phoenix. Knowing how important it is to maintain a healthy body, as a swimmer, I'm compelled to share my experience regarding my father's illness in this book.

Micah Emmanuel Thomas

My YES!

Josiah "Jojo" Martin

August of 2010, I experienced the beginning of a true-life change. While watching over my newborn baby girl, I suddenly was unable to hold down any food or fluids. I got nervous and called her mother to pick her up so I could go to the emergency room. It was there that I found out that my kidney function was at about 15% and that I had a fever of 103. This continued for almost two weeks before they were able to get the fever down. They then did a kidney biopsy, and once all was stable, I was sent home. It took weeks for us to get the results back, but I never imagined the results would be so life-changing.

Going back years before this, I had lost my oldest brother from a seizure he had while preparing to start dialysis. His kidney problems came from FSGS (Focal segmental glomerulosclerosis) which the doctors were now saying that I have! My brother was 29 years old, married, two beautiful young sons, and a son on the way! So, you could imagine the fear and worry that filled the minds of myself and my family! For the next three years, my kidney function would fluctuate. Never too low, but also never in a normal range.

One evening while on tour with Josh Groban and Judith Hill, I began to feel sick and just weird. I went to the urgent care in Florida where we were set to perform that night and found out that my blood pressure was 210/200! They took me to the emergency room where I found out that I had 5% kidney function and would need to start dialysis right away! Because I had no family in Florida, I declined against the doctor's orders. I wanted to be surrounded by people that loved me and with a doctor that truly cared about my well-being before making any major decisions. I found me a wonderful Nephrologist in Atlanta by the name of Dr. Frita Fisher, and I flew back home to begin seeing her for my care. She let me know the severity of my situation and that if I was willing to make the proper lifestyle changes, that I could hold off dialysis for six months!

I began to change my life. I changed my entire diet and lost 100 lbs. I was blessed to have a doctor who had faith that matched mine and together, we worked hard and held off the need for dialysis for six months! Finally, after getting sick and being admitted into the hospital, she told me it was time to start dialysis. Nervous and unsure, I gave everything to God and followed the lead of my Dr. It wasn't as bad as I thought it would be and I had so much support it was overwhelming. We started home peritoneal dialysis where I did dialysis seven days a week 9 hours a night. It wasn't easy, but I didn't complain. Into the second year of this dialysis modality, I got sick so much that the Dr. decided that it was time to move to Hemodialysis in the center. Again, being super nervous, I trusted God and my doctor and went in the center to do dialysis. What a blessing that turned out to be, and how much better I instantly felt!

One night, while in Jacksonville, FL, my best friend and I went for the second time to hear Kirk Franklin in concert. Mainly because it was so amazing the first time in Atlanta, but also because I was so sick that night, I ended up in the hospital for three weeks. So, we decided to go see it again. I was blown away at Gods ultimate plan! During the concert, while ministering a song called, "Intersession," Kirk called me up to sing it with him. That was my first time ever publicly sharing what I was going through with anyone outside my village of trusted friends and family. God met us in a way that I had never experienced before. He listened and comforted me all in one night. He helped me realize that my current journey and all that I would experience to come had nothing to do with me and everything to do with the dying world around me! He reminded me that I was asking Him to use me and that this was what I was saying yes to all these years! I cried tears of hurt, pain, and joy all in one moment. That was the night I gave Him a new yes and vowed to continue to endure as a good soldier!

Realizing that it was almost midnight and a five-hour drive back to Atlanta for dialysis, which was scheduled to start at 5 am, my best friend and I hit the highway to try and get to the clinic on time. I would wake up from time to time to check on her, and she would say, your phone keeps going off. So, I checked my phone and realized that my cousin, who attended the concert as well, had recorded that amazing moment and posted it to Facebook and by the time we were halfway to Atlanta, it had 100,000 views already! I got home right at 5 am, jumped in my car and rushed to the clinic for my 3 ½ hour treatment. You could imagine how tired I was; I fell asleep as soon as they hooked me up to the machine. I woke up just before treatment ended to nurses and other workers saying they were sent my video and had been crying right there in the clinic. I was blown away! So, I checked my phone to see over a million views, and it was less than 12 hrs after the amazing God experience with Kirk Franklin. I had thousands of social media messages and countless text messages, emails, and voicemails. The entire world was praying for me, and I was grateful!

Continuing to travel the world sharing my story and of the goodness of the Lord, there were some bad days, but so many more great days! God filled my life with a joy I hadn't felt in a long time. Ministry from that day forth was expanded not just on stages and in churches, but through messages and many places that I would just casually visit. Countless stories about how people had stopped praying and gave up on God, but after seeing that video their faith was being made new and their prayer life had been restored! I would cry as I marveled at the fruit of my YES! Praying for and talking with people from all walks of life. What a privilege it has been to help other Renal disease patients build their faith to endure and to help newly diagnosed people understand that life wasn't over, and they could not only overcome this but live THROUGH it!!

One Monday after treatment, I got a call from my Emory Transplant coordinator who informed me that they had found a match and not just a match, but it was a living donor...which is exactly what I asked God for! I hung up, rejoiced, cried, and called my family to give them the amazing news. After some final testing and paperwork, I was given my transplant date of August 17, 2018!!! The entire month that I waited, I never knew who the donor was. I was so glad it was happening, I never pushed the issue to find out. That amazing morning, I got up at about 4:15 a.m., woke everyone up like it was Christmas morning, and made a video for social media letting them know for the first time that I had a donor and that I was headed to the hospital for my transplant surgery. Up until then, I had kept that part to myself because I wanted to be praying and staying focused on my still current reality and not the transplant. I wanted to still be in a mental space to help encourage all of those who needed encouragement from me.

I arrived at the hospital at about 5 am and went to register for the surgery. The waiting room had a few people in there but was filling up quickly. I went into the restroom to gather my thoughts and pray by myself. When I came out, my friend Britni was there sitting across the room with her mother and some friends. I heard someone call my name and when I turned around it was her! I said, "What are you doing here so early?" She looked at me, smiled a big smile, and said, "SURPRISE I'M YOUR DONOR!!!" In total shock, we hugged, cried, and laughed about how she never told me she was even trying to be my donor!

I will forever be grateful to God for keeping His word that it would not be unto death! I believe He kept His word with me because I kept mine with Him, pressing through this with everything I had and with a vow to make His name great even amid what some would say were horrific circumstances. I'll forever use my life to glorify His name and spread the word that Jesus is still the absolute answer for us all!

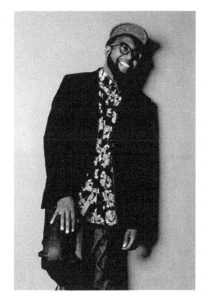

Josiah "JoJo" Martin is the 5th child out of 6, and a 5yr ESRD survivor. Born November 23, 1984, JoJo has achieved many great things in his 34yrs on earth. He's toured all over the world with many amazing artists and musicians, been nominated for numerous awards including a Grammy, and has been the epitome of strength and inspiration for his community and many ESRD survivors all over the world! Currently signed to Morton Records, a label started by Maroon 5's PJ Morton, He is soon to release his first solo project and looks forward to using his life to spread the word about Gods love, organ donations, and ESRD awareness any and everywhere possible!!

PART 4:

It Takes a Village

Babe & Bulldog

Analyn Scott

Let me be clear that Raymond's first term of endearment for me is "Babe." The second is "Bulldog" because he knows that I'm always going to fight to ensure he has the best care. It's important that Raymond is his own biggest advocate, but he jokes around that I know his body & health history better than he does, and that has proven to be very important, especially when he wasn't able to speak for himself.

About a year or so ago Raymond switched to a new primary care physician with the VA, and I joined him for his first appointment. As usual, Raymond deferred most of the questions about his health history to me since I am more thorough and proficient with running down the lengthy and complex timeline. His new physician had to leave the exam room to get some forms off the printer, and when he returned, he had another question that I quickly answered. He looked up from his paper, looked at Raymond and said, "Oh, I get it, you're the sick one, and she's the pain in the butt." I was thinking, "yep, this pain in the butt has helped to keep him alive for 20 years." We still laugh about it today because we didn't believe he intended to be rude, but more so that he has a dry sense of humor. However, it did spark a conversation on the drive home about how many people may not have a health advocate in their corner, especially one that's so outspoken to make sure nothing is missed.

Whether you are healthy or dealing with a chronic illness, it is important that you take charge and be an advocate for your own health. Having a trusted advocate, whether it be a spouse, parent, sibling, child or friend, that can lend their support and help fight for you is very beneficial. Do your research, ask questions, be open and communicate with your physician(s).

Now more than ever this is important because healthcare is often very siloed and rushed and it's easy for important details to fall through the cracks. Don't assume that because it's in the chart, your doctor is aware of your past or current condition. In fact, while we were going over Raymond's health history with his new PCP and mentioned that Raymond currently does home hemodialysis, his physician had a sigh of relief and said, "oh good, from looking at your labs I thought I was going to have to give you bad news about your kidneys." That may have been more of his dry sense of humor, but seriously, Raymond has a pretty long file, so this is one of the reasons we never assume that any of his physicians or specialists have read through it all or are mind readers to know what our top needs and concerns are.

Equally as important for anyone with CKD, ESRD or chronic illness is to have a strong support system. You've likely heard the African proverb, "It takes a village to raise a child," well the same premise rings true in terms of support for individuals and families with kidney disease.

You're not alone. Your village and tribe are larger than you may think.

VILLAGE can be defined as: a self-contained district or community within a town or city, regarded as having features characteristic of village life.

TRIBE can be defined as: A social division in a traditional society consisting of families or communities linked by a social, economic, religious, or blood ties…and…a group of persons having a common character, occupation, or interest.

Raymond and I may live in a village of Phoenix but consider our own "village" to be much more expansive than what is defined as one geographical area on a map. When we look at the support we've given and received it's also not contained in one physical area.

Likewise, the 1in9 Tribe can be found in many villages, cities, states, territories, and countries around the world. We are a diverse tribe made up of people from all walks of life, with one common goal, to beat the drum of hope and change to change the trajectory of kidney disease.

Crowned for Change

Lisa Hedin

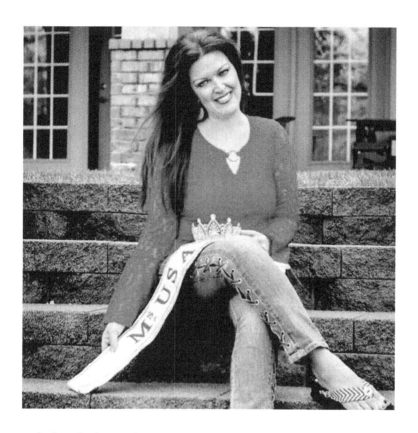

I started this kidney disease journey first, as a family member. I then transformed into making this my career and then became an advocate to spread awareness. I have three points of view on this disease. I will speak to you as a nurse educator, as an advocate and a family member.

During all my years in this field, I will tell you, many people around me have been affected by this disease. Is that a coincidence? No! If you have not been affected by this disease, yet, at some point, you will be, by either yourself or someone close to you in the progression of kidney disease. I have so many friends and family members who will call me with their lab values for me to look over. Age does not discriminate against this disease as I have identified some of my friends in their 40's and 50's in stage 3 kidney disease. What is even more mind-boggling is that their doctor did not even address it with them at their appointment. That is where the 1in9 tribe comes in. We are here to educate and make you aware.

It's so important to catch this early so you can slow down the progression and take the appropriate measures to keep your kidneys from reaching the last stage, stage 5. It is possible for you to slow down the progression and live a relatively symptom-free life if caught early enough. The kidneys are very hearty organs, and you only need 10% function of one kidney to sustain life.

During my 20+ years of specializing in kidney disease as an RN, most of my patients did not know that they had kidney disease until they were in their final stages. To me, that is unacceptable since there are five stages of kidney disease and there are simple tests for healthcare professionals to do to identify this silent killer. Often, it is missed, when the whole picture is not looked at in full. In most cases, kidney disease just doesn't happen overnight. I had a physician once say, "It's like an old tree that is dying. The leaves start dying one by one until the whole tree is dead." Same with kidney disease, usually its years of progression.

As a family member, imagine, not knowing anything about kidney disease, and being uneducated about the treatment. A machine is wheeled into an intensive care unit. You see your loved one's blood being pumped outside the body, then pushed through an artificial kidney, and then pushed back into the body with a large intravenous line going into the neck of your loved one. All of this, while nurses and doctors are tackling blood pressure issues, heart rates and stabilizing the symptoms that a new dialysis patient may encounter. It's traumatic for family members and patients. This is something that can easily be avoided by the proper testing and education before becoming a patient getting to the last stages of kidney disease.

I watched my dad go through this while in an intensive care unit, unresponsive and trying to stay alive during his first few dialysis treatments. I was a young nursing student in my early 20's and that is how I got introduced to the kidneys. No book in nursing school prepared for that scenario and what I was going to see while my dad fought for his life. It was hard on my family to witness this, and I knew right then and there that my career was going to be focused around kidney disease.

I always say this when I do public speaking. "The most painful experiences in life, will most times become your purpose in life."

My dad at the time had acute kidney failure.

There is a difference between chronic and acute kidney disease. Most cases it's chronic kidney disease where the kidneys die slowly. Let me explain the differences between acute and chronic:

Acute

Acute kidney injury (AKI) is a sudden episode of kidney failure or kidney damage that happens within a few hours or a few days. AKI causes a build-up of waste products in your blood and makes it hard for your kidneys to keep the right balance of fluid in your body. AKI can also affect other organs such as the brain, heart, and lungs. Acute kidney injury is common in patients who are in the hospital, in intensive care units, and especially in older adults.

(Reference: National Kidney Foundation - *https://www.kidney.org/atoz/content/AcuteKidneyInjury*)

- Too little urine leaving the body
- Swelling in legs, ankles, and around the eyes
- Fatigue or tiredness
- Shortness of breath
- Confusion
- Nausea
- Seizures or coma in severe cases
- • Chest pain or pressure

In some cases, AKI causes no symptoms and is only found through other tests done by your healthcare provider.

Chronic

Chronic kidney disease includes conditions that damage your kidneys and decrease their ability to keep you healthy by doing the jobs listed. If kidney disease gets worse, wastes can build to high levels in your blood, and make you feel sick. You may develop complications like high blood pressure, anemia (low blood count), weak bones, poor nutritional health, and nerve damage. Also, kidney disease increases your risk of having heart and blood vessel disease. These problems may happen slowly over a long period. Chronic kidney disease may be caused by diabetes, high blood pressure, and other disorders. Early detection and treatment can often keep chronic kidney disease from getting worse. When kidney disease progresses, it may eventually lead to kidney failure, which requires dialysis or a kidney transplant to maintain life.

30 million American adults have CKD, and millions of others are at increased risk.

- Early detection can help prevent the progression of kidney disease to kidney failure.

- Heart disease is the major cause of death for all people with CKD.
- Glomerular filtration rate (GFR) is the best estimate of kidney function.
- Hypertension causes CKD and CKD causes hypertension.
- Persistent proteinuria (protein in the urine) means CKD is present.
- High-risk groups include those with diabetes, hypertension and family history of kidney failure.
- African Americans, Hispanics, Pacific Islanders, American Indians and Seniors are at increased risk.
- • Two simple tests can detect CKD: blood pressure, urine albumin and serum creatinine.

End Stage Renal Disease (ESRD) is the 5th and final stage of kidney disease. Unfortunately, there is a lack in education to give patients all the options on the modality for kidney disease. We are getting better, but we have a long way to go. Patients need to take a proactive approach with their physician, nurse and social worker to choose the modality that best fits their needs and lifestyles. The following are a list of the modalities that are available here in the United States (Reference: National Kidney Foundation)

Hemodialysis:

In hemodialysis, an artificial kidney (hemodialyzer) is used to remove waste and extra chemicals and fluid from your blood. To get your blood into the artificial kidney, the doctor needs to make an access (entrance) into your blood vessels. This is done by minor surgery to your arm or leg.

Sometimes, an access is made by joining an artery to a vein under your skin to make a bigger blood vessel called a fistula.

However, if your blood vessels are not adequate for a fistula, the doctor may use a soft plastic tube to join an artery and a vein under your skin. This is called a graft.

Occasionally, an access is made by means of a narrow plastic tube, called a catheter, which is inserted into a large vein in your neck. This type of access may be temporary but is sometimes used for long-term treatment.

Peritoneal Dialysis:

In this type of dialysis, your blood is cleaned inside your body. The doctor will do surgery to place a plastic tube called a catheter into your abdomen (belly) to make an access. During the treatment, your abdominal area (called the peritoneal cavity) is slowly filled with dialysate through the catheter. The blood stays in the arteries and veins that line your peritoneal cavity. Extra fluid and waste products are drawn out of your blood and into the dialysate.

Nocturnal Hemodialysis:

Nocturnal means occurring at night. Nocturnal dialysis is a slower, longer hemodialysis treatment that takes place at night while you sleep. This longer treatment is for six to eight hours, three times or more a week. You can do nocturnal dialysis at home or at a dialysis center that has a nocturnal dialysis program.

Home Hemodialysis

This dialysis is essentially the same as hemodialysis except it is done at home. The machine is generally a little simpler to operate. When at home, it is desirable to have a home helper who will go through the training with you.

Kidney Transplant:

A kidney transplant is an operation that places a healthy kidney from another person into your body. The kidney may come from someone who has died or from a living donor who may be a close relative, spouse or friend. It can even come from someone who wishes to donate a kidney to anyone in need of a transplant. However, a kidney transplant is a treatment, not a cure, and it is important to care for the new kidney with the same care as before receiving the transplant

I felt that I had to switch my gears a bit and start advocating more and preventing this disease. As I have been on this journey with kidney disease, I've always worked on the back end taking care of sick patients, and I realized that I needed to be on the front end and catch these patients early before it got them sick.

When I was crowned Ms. North Carolina back in 2015, I joined forces with the National Kidney Foundation in the Carolinas to bring awareness to this disease. I knew this was an opportunity to make a big impact in getting the word out. I made several media appearances, and we raised close to $20,000.00 to get free screenings and more education out to the public. We have helped several people who were already in the disease process and had no idea.

I was then named Ms. USA, awarded that title based on the humanitarian efforts I put forth in bringing awareness to this disease. It was surprising to be informed by the Ms. USA and Ms. America organization that this was the first-time kidney disease was selected as a platform. Let me put this into perspective for you on why this is so important to me and should be important to all of you. More people die of kidney disease than breast cancer every year. Astounding huh? We have so much marketing about breast cancer, and you see so little about kidney disease. This is such an easy fix with a very simple test where we can stop this from being an epidemic in our country

I take this very seriously as I have traveled all over the United States and hear the same story over and over from patients and family members "We were shocked he/she even had kidney disease, and from what we found out is that the kidneys were declining for years when our lab work was evaluated". The is an epidemic in our country, and I stress to all people I meet that you must take control over your own care. Be proactive in telling the doctors you want to see certain lab tests such as BUN, CREAT, GFR and a urinalysis to check for protein in the urine. It's that simple and we must educate the public.

The National Kidney Foundation offers free screening in your area. I urge you to take advantage of these free screenings.

I do still work on the back end of this disease as an educator for a medical manufacturing company that manufactures dialysis equipment, but I spend a lot of time on the front-end bringing awareness to this deadly disease. A disease that can be managed if caught early. Through awareness, we can create a major shift to help more people prevent or at least catch this disease early. That would drastically reduce the number of people who would need to see me on the back end. I welcome the fact that I could be unemployed because we beat this epidemic!

Lisa is a registered nurse that has dedicated her career to kidney disease since 1994. With her role as Ms. North Carolina America and Ms. USA, she aligned with the National Kidney Foundation-Carolinas and made several TV appearances to educate the public on kidney disease. With her many event appearances, she has teamed with local celebrities, sports teams and music legends to raise money for research & awareness.

Lisa was the former Ms. North Carolina and in 2015 she won the "Woman of Distinction" award. The Ms. America pageant organization felt she deserved the honor because she represented beauty, intelligence and the humanitarian efforts of what the American woman represents. All her efforts have been directed towards kidney disease awareness.

Lisa is a senior clinical educator for a major innovative company that manufactures products to help those with kidney disease. Just this past year in Las Vegas, Lisa was honored to receive a prestigious award of "Clinical Educator of the Year"

Lisa is a mother to a teenage boy who is the love of her life and likes spending her free time at the gym, boxing or hot yoga. She is originally from Pittsburgh, Pennsylvania and her Pittsburgh sports teams are near and dear to her heart.

Slow It Down CKD

Gail Rae-Garwood

My name is Gail Rae-Garwood. I like to think of myself as an average older woman with two adult daughters, a fairly recent husband, and a very protective dog. But I'm not. What makes me a little different is that I have Chronic Kidney Disease…just like the estimated 30 million or 15% of the adult population in the United States. Unlike 96% of those in the early stages of the disease, I know my kidneys are not functioning well.

Once upon a time, a long, long time ago, before I'd ever heard the word nephrology, I paid no attention to my kidneys. I had just a vague idea of where they were located because I had big brothers. Every time they watched boxing, one or the other of them would yell, "Oh! Right in the kidneys!" when one guy hit the other on the back, sort of near the waist. My mother attempted to feed us kidney beans once or twice, but three voices chorusing the 1950's equivalent of "Uh, gross!" was enough to convince her they weren't that necessary. My father had a friend who'd moved up in the world and had a kidney shaped pool. Of course, I never had a bird's eye view of that as a child. So, we were a family pretty much ignorant about kidneys.

When I grew up, I never let my children watch boxing; it was too violent. I never even tried to feed them kidney beans, probably due to some residual abhorrence left over from my own childhood. I had no friends with kidney shaped pools, but I had flown in an airplane and could recognize one if we were flying low. That was the sum total of my kidney education. I didn't even recall if they were covered in high school biology. My daughters, now grown women, said they were, but I didn't remember anything about that.

I was blindsided over a decade ago. That's when I started seeing a new doctor solely because she was both on my insurance plan and so much closer to home than the one, I'd been seeing. It seems everything is at least half an hour away in Arizona; her office wasn't. As a diligent primary care physician, she ordered a whole battery of tests to verify what she found in my files which, by the way, contained a kidney function reading (called the GFR) of 39%. That was something I'd never been told about.

39%. I'd been a high school teacher for 35 years at that point. If a student had scored 39% on a test, we would have talked and talked until we had gotten to the root of the problem that caused such a low score. No one talked to me about my low kidney function until I changed doctors.

"That's not normal," said my new doctor as she looked at my blood test results.

I made the supreme effort of tearing my eyes away from the height and weight chart to ask, "What's not normal?"

"Your GFR," she told me. I looked at her blankly. (In retrospect, I can understand how hard it probably was for her not to laugh at my empty eyes and a face without a shred of interest showing on it.) I said nothing. She said nothing.

Finally, I asked, "What's that?" She gave me a simple explanation with no indication that I should panic in any way, but of course I did.

"It's what! It's below normal? My kidneys aren't functioning to full capacity? Why wasn't I told? What do I do now? How do I fix the problem? I want them at 100%."

Her voice rose over mine in a steady, sure manner. "This does not mean there is a problem. It means you must go to a specialist to see if there really is a problem."

"Oh." I didn't believe her, but she not only talked, she had me in a nephrologist's (kidney and hypertension specialist) office the next day. That's when I started worrying. Who gets an appointment with a specialist the very next day? I was diagnosed at stage 3; there are only 5 stages. I had to start working to slow down the progression in the decline of my kidney function immediately.

I read just about every book I could find concerning this problem. Surprisingly, very few books dealt with the early or moderate stages of the disease. Yet these are the stages when CKD patients are most shocked, confused, and maybe even depressed—and the stages at which they have a workable chance of doing something to slow down the progression in the decline of their kidney function.

This first nephrologist might have been reassuring, but I'll never know. I was terrified; he was patriarchal. All I heard was, "I'll take care of your kidneys. You just do as I say," or something to that effect.

Nope, wrong doctor for me. I wanted to know how medication, diet, exercise and other lifestyle changes could help. I didn't want to be told what to do without an explanation as to why… and when I couldn't get an explanation that was acceptable to me, I started researching. (More about that later.) You see, I'd already had a terrific Dad who'd known better than to ask me to give up control of myself. I didn't need a doctor assuming his role…especially in a way I resented.

Nephrologist switch. The new one was much better for me. He explained again and again until I understood, and he put up with a lot of verbal abuse when this panicky new patient wasn't getting answers as quickly as she wanted them. Luckily for me, he graciously accepted my apology.

After talking to the nephrologist, I began to realize just how serious this disease was and started to wonder why my previous nurse practitioner had not caught this. When I asked her why, she responded, "It was inconclusive testing." Sure, it was. Because she never ordered the GFR tested; that had been incidental! I feel there's no sense crying over spilled milk (or destroyed nephrons, in this case), but I wonder how much more of my kidney function I could have preserved if I'd known about my CKD earlier.

According to the Mayo Clinic, there are 13 early signs of chronic kidney disease. I never experienced any of them, not even one. While I did have high blood pressure, it wasn't uncontrollable which is one of the early signs. Many, like me, never experienced any noticeable symptoms. Unfortunately, many, like me, may have had high blood pressure (hypertension) for years before CKD was diagnosed. Yet, high blood pressure and diabetes are the two leading causes of CKD. I find it confusing that uncontrollable high blood pressure may be an early sign of CKD, but hypertension itself is the second leading cause of CKD.

Here's the part about my researching. I was so mystified about what was happening and why it was happening that I began an extensive course of research. My nephrologists did explain what everything meant (I think), but I was still too shocked to understand what they were saying. I researched diagnoses, descriptions of tests, test results, doctors' reports, you name it. Slowly, it began to make sense, but that understanding only led to more questions and more research.

You've probably already guessed that my world changed during that first appointment. I began to excuse myself for rest periods each day when I went back East for a slew of family affairs right after. I counted food groups and calories at these celebrations that summer. And I used all the errand running associated with them as an excuse to speed walk wherever I went and back so I could fit in my exercise. Ah, but that was just the beginning.

My high blood pressure had been controlled for 20 years at that time, but what about my diet? I had no clue there was such a thing as a kidney diet until the nutritionist explained it to me. I'm a miller's granddaughter and ate anything – and I do mean anything - with grain in it: breads, muffins, cakes, croissants, all of it. I also liked lots of chicken and fish… not the five ounces per day I'm limited to now.

The nutritionist explained to me how hard protein is on the kidneys…as is phosphorous…and potassium…and, of course, sodium. Out went my daily banana—too high in potassium. Out went restaurant burgers—larger than my daily allowance of protein. Chinese food? Pizza? Too high in sodium. I embraced an entirely new way of eating because it was one of the keys to keeping my kidneys functioning in stage 3.

I was in a new food world. I'd already known about restricting sodium because I had high blood pressure, but these other things? I had to keep a list of which foods contain them, how much was in each of these foods, and a running list of how much of each I had during the day, so I knew when I reached my limit for that day.

Another critical piece of slowing down CKD is medication. I was already taking meds to lower my blood pressure when I was first diagnosed with CKD. Two more prescriptions have been added to this in the last decade: a diuretic that lowers my body's absorption of salt to help prevent fluid from building up in my body (edema), and a drug that widens the blood vessels by relaxing them. I take another drug for my brand-new diabetes. (Bye-bye, sugars and most carbs.) The funny thing is now my favorite food is salad with extra virgin olive oil and balsamic vinegar. I never thought that would happen: I was a chocoholic!

Exercise, something I loved until my arthritis got in the way, was also important. I was a dancer. Wasn't that enough? Uh-uh, I had to learn about cardio and strength training exercise, too. It was no longer acceptable to be pleasantly plumb. My kidneys didn't need the extra work. Hello to weights, walking, and a stationary bike. I think I took sleep for granted before CKD, too, and I now make it a point to get a good night's sleep. A sleep apnea device improved my sleep—and my kidney function rose.

I realized I needed to rest, too. Instead of giving a lecture, running to an audition, and coming home to meet a deadline, I slowly started easing off until I didn't feel like I was running on empty all the time. The result was that I ended up graciously retiring from both acting and teaching at a local college, which gave me more time to work on my CKD awareness advocacy.

But I had to be oh-so-vigilant with other medical practitioners. One summer I had four different infections and had to quickly research the medications prescribed in the emergency room. One hospital insisted I could take sulfa drugs because I was only stage 2 at the time. My nephrologist disagreed. They also prescribed a pain killer with acetaminophen in it, another no-no for us. I didn't return to them when I developed the other infections.

My experience demonstrates that you can slow down CKD. I was diagnosed at stage 3 and I am still there, over a decade later. It takes knowledge, commitment and discipline—but it can be done, and it's worth the effort. I'm sneaking up on 72 now and know this is where I want to spend my energy for the rest of my life: chronic kidney disease awareness advocacy. I think it's just that important.

At the time of my diagnosis, I was a college instructor. My favorite course to teach was Research Writing. I was also a writer with an Academic Certificate in Creative Non-Fiction and a bunch of publications under my belt. It occurred to me that I couldn't be the only one who had no clue what this new-to-me disease was and how to handle living with it. I knew how to research, and I knew how to write, so why not share what I learned?

I wasn't sure of what had to be done to share or how to do it. I learned by trial and error. People were so kind in teaching me, pointing out what might work better, even suggesting others that might be interested in what I was doing. I love people.

I'd written quite a few how to(s), study guides, articles, and literary guides so the writing was not new to me. I asked for suggestions as to what to do with my writing and that's when I learned about unscrupulous, price gouging vanity publishers. I'm still paying for the unwitting mistakes I made, but they were learning experiences.

My less-than-stellar experience with being diagnosed and the first nephrologist are what prompted me to write *What Is It and How Did I Get It? Early Stage Chronic Kidney Disease.* Why, I wondered, should any new CKD patient be as terrified as I was? Of course, I constantly remind my readers that I'm not a doctor and they need to consult their nephrologists or renal dietitians before making any changes to their regiment.

I didn't feel…well, done with sharing or researching once I finished the book, so I began writing a weekly blog: SlowItDownCKD. Well, that and because a nephrologist in India told me he wanted his newly diagnosed patients to read my book, but most of them couldn't afford the bus fare to the clinic, much less a book. I published each chapter as a blog post. The nephrologist translated my posts, printed them and distributed them to his patients—who took the printed copies back to their communities.

It would work! But first I had to teach myself how to blog. I made some boo-boos and lost a bunch of blogs until I got it figured out. So why do I keep blogging? There always seems to be more to share about CKD. Each week, I wonder what I'll write…and the ideas keep coming.

I now have readers in something like 106 different countries who ask me questions I hadn't even thought of. I research for them and respond with a blog post, reminding them to speak with their nephrologists and/or renal nutritionists before taking any action… and that I'm not a doctor.

The blog has won several awards. Basically, that's because I write in a reader friendly manner. After all, what good is all my researching if no one understands what I'm writing? Non-tech savvy readers asked if I could print the blogs; hence, the birth of the *SlowItDownCKD* series of books.

Some people think *SlowItDownCKD* is a business; it's not. Some think it's a profit maker; it's not. So, what is it you ask? It's a vehicle for spreading awareness of Chronic Kidney Disease and whatever goes along with the disease. Why do I do it? Because I had no idea what it was, nor how I might have prevented the disease, nor how to deal with it effectively once I was diagnosed. I couldn't stand the thought of others being in the same position.

One of my daughters taught me about social media. What??? You could post whatever you wanted to? And Facebook wasn't the only way to reach the public at large? Hello, LinkedIn. A friend who is a professional photographer asked me why I wasn't using my fun photography habit to promote awareness. What??? You could do that? Enter Instagram. My step-daughters love Pinterest. That got me to thinking and suddenly *SlowItDownCKD* had a Pinterest account. Then someone I met at a conference casually mentioned she offers Twitter workshops. What kind of workshops? She showed me how to use Twitter to raise CKD awareness.

When I was diagnosed back in 2008, there weren't that many reader friendly books on anything having to do with CKD. Since then, more and more books of this type have been published. I'm laughing along with you, but I don't mean just *SlowItDownCKD 2011*, *SlowItDownCKD 2012* (These two were The Book of Blogs: Moderate Stage Chronic Kidney Disease, Part 1, until I realized how unwieldy both the book and the title were – another learning experience), *SlowItDownCKD 2013*, *SlowItDownCKD 2014* (These two were formerly The Book of Blogs: Moderate Stage Chronic Kidney Disease, Part 2), *SlowItDownCKD 2015*, *SlowItDownCKD 2016*, and *SlowItDownCKD 2017*. By the way, I'm already working on *SlowItDownCKD 2018*. Each book contains the blogs for that year.

I include guest blogs or book review blogs to get a taste of the currently available CKD news. For example, 1in9 guest blogged this year. Books such as Dr. Mandip S. Kang's, *The Doctor's Kidney Diets* (which also contains so much non-dietary information that we - as CKD patients - need to know), and Drs. Raymond R. Townsend and Debbie L. Cohen's *100 Questions & Answers about Kidney Disease and Hypertension.*

I miss my New York daughter and she misses me, so we sometimes have coffee together separately. She has a cup of coffee and I do at the same time. It's not like being together in person, but it's something. You can find support the same way via Facebook Chronic Kidney Disease Support Groups. Some of these groups are:

- Chronic Kidney Disease Awareness
- Chronic Kidney Disease in India
- CKD (Kidney Failure) Support Group International
- Dialysis & Kidney Disease
- Friends Sharing Positive Chronic Kidney Disease
- I Hate Dialysis
- Kidney Disease Diet Ideas and Help
- Kidney Disease Ideas and Diets1
- Kidney Disease is not a Joke

- Kidney Disease, Dialysis, and Transplant
- Kidney Warriors Foundation
- Kidneys and Vets
- Mani Trust
- Mark's Private Kidney Disease Group
- P2P
- People on Dialysis
- Sharing your Kidney Journey
- Stage 3 'n 4 Kidneybeaners Gathering Place
- The Transplant Community Outreach
- UK Kidney Support
- Women's Renal Failure
- Wrap Up Warm for Kidney Disease

What I hit repeatedly in the blogs is that diabetes is the foremost cause of CKD with hypertension as the second most common cause. Simple blood and urine tests can uncover your CKD – if you're part of the unlucky 96% of those in the early stages of the disease who don't know they have it.

Each time I research, I'm newly amazed at how much there is to learn about CKD…and how many tools you have at your disposal to help slow it down. Diet is the obvious one. But if you smoke or drink, stop, or at least cut down. If you don't exercise, start. Adequate, good quality sleep is another tool. Don't underestimate rest either; you're not being lazy when you rest, you're preserving whatever kidney function you have left. I am not particularly a pill person, but if there's a medication prescribed that will slow down the gradual decline of my kidney function, I'm all for it.

I was surprised to discover that writing my *SlowItDownCKD* book series, maintaining a blog, Facebook page, Twitter, Instagram, and

Pinterest accounts of the same name are not enough for me for me to spread the word about CKD screening and education. I'm determined to change this since I feel so strongly that NO ONE should have this disease and not be aware of it.

That's why I've brought CKD awareness to every community that would have me: coffee shops, Kiwanis Clubs, independent bookstores, senior citizen centers, guest blogging for the likes of The American Kidney Fund and The National Kidney Foundation, being interviewed by publications like the Wall Street Journal's Health Matters, The Center for Science in The Public Interest, and The United Federation of Teachers' New York Teacher, and on podcasts such as The Renal Diet Headquarters, Online with Andrea, The Edge Podcast, Working with Chronic Illness, and Improve Your Kidney Health.

I've been very serious about sharing about CKD before it advances to end stage…meaning dialysis. To that end, I gathered a team for the National Kidney Foundation of Arizona Kidney Walk one year. Another year, I organized several meetings at the Salt River Pima-Maricopa Indian Community. Education is vital since so many people are unaware, they even have the disease.

You can slow down the progression of the decline of kidney function. I have been spending a lot of time on my health and I'm happy to say it's been paying off. There are five stages. I've stayed at the middle one for over a decade despite having both high blood pressure and diabetes. That's what this is about. People don't know about CKD. They get diagnosed. They think they're going to die. Everybody dies, but it doesn't have to be of CKD. I am downright passionate about people knowing this.

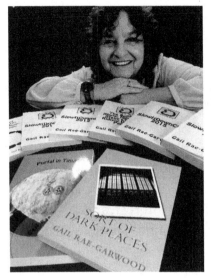

Ms. Rae-Garwood's writing started out as a means to an end for a single parent with two children and a need for more income than her career as a NYC teacher afforded. Gail retired from both college teaching and acting - after a bit of soul searching about where her CKD limited energy would be best spent - early in 2013. Since her diagnose, Ms. Rae-Garwood writes most often about Chronic Kidney Disease, although she does write fiction. She has a three-time award winning weekly blog about this topic at *http://gailraegarwood.wordpress.com* and social media accounts as *@SlowItDownCKD*.

Faith and Basketball

Ericka Downey

I've been a part of the college basketball family for more than a decade. My husband, Mark Downey, is the head basketball coach at Northeastern State University in Tahlequah, Oklahoma. Together, his career has moved us six times. We have two beautiful children. Bryce is 13 and Drew, 7. This is my personal journey on how we gave back to the sport that has given so much to us.

One winter day, I sat in my messy closet floor procrastinating at the task at hand. To be frank, it was a disaster. I'm a medical device rep with a territory that covered four states. I traveled a lot. Often, I would come home from one business trip, discard my luggage in my closet, grab a second piece and depart for the next. Consecutive weeks of this habit starred back at me on December 16, 2017. It was a Saturday. Instead of attacking the project head on I grabbed my cell phone on the floor beside me. This is where the real story begins.

As I sat there scrolling through Twitter, a storyline caught my attention. The headline from a Dallas Morning News Article specifically. It read, "Former Texas A&M, Texas Tech, Kentucky basketball coach Billy Gillispie in urgent need of a kidney transplant." I read the whole story multiple times, each time the feeling building from the last. I knew the name Billy Gillispie, but most importantly I knew I needed to act.

I grew up in church and still find my faith as a source of strength. My grandparents adopted me and my older brother as toddlers. I was in the 5th grade when I became a Christian. Like many, I have at times questioned God. But not today. Not that day. God's prompting to be a willing donor was so clear as I rushed to find answers on the living donor process that afternoon.

The article said that Coach Gillispie would be seeking treatment at Mayo Clinic in Rochester, Minnesota. Their website was my first stop. That is where I came across the user-friendly online living donor application. I completed it on the spot without hesitation. One of the questions was "Do you have an intended recipient?" Name_____, Date of Birth_____. I knew the name Billy Gillispie, but I didn't know him. I knew he was a talented basketball coach, and that he had a brief stint as the leader of Big Blue Nation (Kentucky Wildcats.) Being raised in Arkansas, you have one team, The Arkansas Razorbacks. Essentially, we were once rivals, SEC rivals.

Because I didn't know Billy Gillispie, I didn't know if Billy was his given name. I also didn't know his birthday, but I googled it. I didn't know his blood type or any of his contact info. None of that mattered. I knew the answers on that health questionnaire. That's what counted. I also continued to pray for guidance in the process. My personality can be very spontaneous. I know that about me. My husband often reminds me, but this seemed different. It wasn't just a big idea or another project. I was going to see this through.

Remember that messy, unorganized closet? It was still there. I hit submit and called the 1-800 number on the Mayo Clinic website. After all the googled answers, I still had questions. Since it was the weekend, I got a recorded message. I realized I had done all I could do for the day. I retweeted the story for good measure just in case someone else read it and felt the call to help. Then, I cleaned.

This is where the self-doubt and fear sat in. "Oh, my goodness," I thought. I just did all of this without speaking to my husband. What will he think? What will he say? My Father-in-law passed away in 2009 after a three-year battle with renal failure. I didn't understand his fight

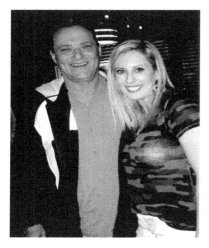
Erika Downey & Billy Gillispie

then. Mark is twelve years older than me and was born when his parents were in their mid-40s. I just thought his body was aging. My father-in-law was on daily in-home dialysis. My mother-in-law, then in her 80s, was his sole caregiver. The machine and process were complicated, but she took pride in learning to care for him. He died in June, and Mark and I married in August the same year.

As you can see, I had a lot on my mind. I chose to meditate through those thoughts privately with God until I could get clarity. It wasn't until the next day when I spoke to my husband about my actions. I walked into the living room on Sunday after church. He was lying on the couch watching tv. I asked him about Coach Gillispie. "Were you aware of his health issues?" I asked. After sharing the story and that I felt called to donate, he responded. "You're crazy!" We laughed. You see, he knew that when he married me. It didn't stop him then, and he knew that very moment my mind was made up.

Monday rolled around, and I was back on the phone with Mayo Clinic. Because there are laws protecting patient information, I couldn't get much information about Coach Gillispie. All they would tell me is they didn't have a Billy Gillispie on the waiting list. How could that be? I called every week to "check back" as the living donor nurse recommended. There wasn't any news.

A month later I was traveling to Las Vegas for a work meeting when I received a private message on Twitter. It read:

"Hi, Ericka. My name is Josh Mills and I am very close with Coach Gillispie. I was his assistant last year at Ranger and at Texas Tech. He doesn't have twitter account, but I showed him your tweets and how much you are trying to help him. He wanted to thank you, could you give him a call or shoot him a text please?"

The message included his phone number. This was the breakthrough I needed. I was in flight and couldn't connect immediately but texted him when I landed. He was, as you can imagine, incredibly thankful and kind. He hadn't been approved for transplant pending formal testing. He gave me the dates of the scheduled visit and said the transplant process should ramp up quickly after that. Coach Gillispie was originally treated with high blood pressure in 2012 at the Mayo Clinic. He never consistently took his medication resulting in irreversible damage. Stage 4 kidney failure to be exact. He was six months or less away from dialysis. In his words, "he never felt sick." Ladies and gentlemen let me introduce you to the silent killer, kidney disease.

He was right. Three weeks later, I received the blood testing kit. I took it to my local lab, completed the blood draw and returned overnight. On February 19, I got the call. It was my living donor nurse, Lisa King. "Ericka, do you have a few minutes to talk?" My labs showed we were a match. I needed to do a 24-hour urine collection and make my way to Minnesota for extensive testing to ensure I was healthy enough to donate. The first available date was the last week of March.

The last week of March was already circled on my calendar. That was the same week as the Final Four basketball tournament in San Antonio. I planned to go Monday-Wednesday for testing in Minnesota then travel straight to the Final Four. It's a yearly post season trip for my husband and me. The NABC (National Association of Basketball Coaches) convention always coincides with the Final Four. It's an opportunity for us to reunite with our friends in the profession and celebrate our successes from the basketball season. My family would meet me there.

I went through all the required tests without any issues. My overseeing nephrologist said they always find something. It was no different with me. The CT scan with contrast revealed a fatty tumor on my right kidney between my adrenal gland and kidney. It was so small that it was hard to see on the images. And my iron was low. I walked away with an all clear from my medical team and a prescription for iron.

I think one of the most reassuring things during the process is having a completely separate medical team from the recipient. My team knew nothing about Coach Gillispie. His team knew nothing about me. They want to keep the donor's assessment without bias. I felt that my health was always the priority. Our medical teams met on Thursday morning to review the cases for the first time. After all medical information was reviewed, we were approved for surgery.

By this time, I had arrived in San Antonio with my family. I called Coach Gillispie to share the news with him. He needed to call to schedule the surgery, so we didn't have a date yet. I host a party every year on Friday at the Final Four for coaches and their families who have worked with us. Social media gives us a way to stay in touch

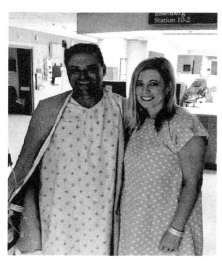

throughout the year but having the opportunity to catch up in person is so important to Mark and me. I had invited Coach Gillispie. At this point, I had been through the entire living donor process, and I had yet to meet my recipient. We met that Friday night at our yearly event. Coach had talked to his medical team, and they gave us the first available surgery date of April 24, 2018. We took it.

We flew to Rochester, MN on the Sunday prior to our surgery. I had to repeat labs on Monday to make sure my health had not deteriorated in the month since the last ones. It was finally surgery day. I was determined to walk to his room after surgery, but that didn't happen. I got about halfway there before I collapsed. My blood pressure dropped, and my nurse caught me with a wheelchair. That was disappointing. My emotions were all over the place those three days in the hospital. I struggled to get out of bed most days. I slept a lot and cried even more.

Coach Gillispie would stop by my room on his daily 4-mile walks around the hospital wing. That was so confusing. Why was I struggling? I didn't understand. As I follow other kidney transplant stories, this seems to come up a lot. I was a healthy person, made sick. He was very ill, and the new kidney was working to purify the toxins out of his body. He felt better than he had in a very long time. In addition to the kidney improvement, he was on a lot of medication that increased his energy. The best advice I got during this time was "listen to your body."

I was discharged from the hospital on Thursday but was required to stay close to the hospital until Sunday. Coach was discharged on Friday. He needed to stick around for three weeks. I didn't experience any complications. I got through the procedure and recovery without the use of opioids. In my career field, I have seen the negative effects of opioids and requested to stay away from them. The shoulder pain caught me off guard. The procedure to remove a donor kidney is called hand-assisted, laparoscopic nephrectomy. To separate the internal organs, they pump the patient full of gases. It takes weeks to work itself out of the body. The gases get trapped in the upper torso and shoulders causing extreme discomfort. Medication doesn't help with that. I found walking and heat were my friends.

It's been over a year since our journey began. In September we reunited in Rochester for our 6-month follow up. The kidney has made a home with Coach Gillispie with no signs of rejection. My labs are very close to returning to a normal level. I never stop worrying about him and his health. I'm certain he never stops worrying about me. That's how it will always be. Rejection can occur at any point, but with advances in medicine rejection rates improve over time.

Coach Gillispie is back on the sidelines this season after a forced sabbatical due to his rapid health decline last year. He is the head basketball coach at Ranger College, a junior college in Ranger, TX. The team is currently 14-2 and ranked in the top 10 in junior college rankings. He's in his rightful place; living his best life. God is faithful.

PART 5:

Medical Tribe

Vantage Point: A Nephrologist's View of Kidney Disease

Elise J. Barney, DO

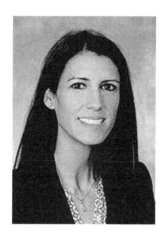

Why do I care about my kidneys? Maybe I am biased, (ok I'm definitely biased, but hear me out) but I have found the kidneys to be the most intricate finely-tuned machine in the body. They do the great balancing act of keeping the body in perfect metabolic harmony on a daily basis.

The kidneys regulate water, salt, electrolytes such as calcium, magnesium, phosphorous, your pH, and even glucose! They secrete a hormone called erythropoietin that tells your bone marrow to make red blood cells, so you don't get anemic. They secrete hormones to keep your blood pressure normal. They metabolize drugs and excrete toxins and waste in the urine. Without proper kidney function, waste and fluid can build up and cause damage to the body. It can lead to heart disease and increase the risk of heart attack or stroke. Yes, the simple act of urination we take for granted every day is one of the most important functions of our body and without it, we could die.

What are the symptoms of kidney disease? Surprisingly, due to the body's ability to accommodate and tolerate decreased kidney function, there are not many symptoms until kidney disease has advanced significantly. However, some symptoms to look for include swelling, nausea, itchiness, and changes in urination, such as foamy urine or blood in the urine. High blood pressure can also be a sign of kidney disease. Some persons with diabetes sustain improved blood glucose control and even hypoglycemia (low blood sugars) from failing kidneys because the diabetes drugs and insulin are not getting fully metabolized. The best way to know how your kidneys are functioning is by getting routine blood and urine tests yearly. If one is at increased risk for kidney disease, these tests should be done even more frequently.

What exactly is chronic kidney disease? While the term chronic kidney disease (CKD) is a general term used to describe a decrease in filtration of the kidneys over a minimum period of 3 months, it encompasses a broad pathology of clinical syndromes. Kidney disease comes in all shapes and sizes. It affects all types of people worldwide, with a higher prevalence in females, older patients, African-Americans, Pacific Islanders, and Latinos. The number one cause of CKD in the U.S. is diabetes, and number two is hypertension (high blood pressure). Other causes include autoimmune diseases like systemic lupus erythematosus (SLE), glomerulonephritis from infections or other immune-related causes, and genetic diseases such as polycystic kidney disease and Alport's syndrome. There are also a growing number of patients with kidney disease from unrecovered acute kidney injury or failure, meaning an abrupt or sudden dysfunction of the kidneys.

Acute kidney injury can be caused by shock or severe, overwhelming infections in the body, severe dehydration and heat exhaustion, kidney stones, and bladder obstruction, heart or liver failure, and medications. Medications that are harmful to the kidneys include chemotherapy drugs, some antibiotics and even over the counter medications and supplements like Ibuprofen. Procedures such as heart surgery and contrast dye from catheter interventions and CT scans can also lead to acute kidney injury.

The silver lining is that acute kidney injury is typically thought of as temporary and patients can recover, even if they require dialysis. The kidneys can essentially "bounce back" from damage if it is short-lived. Sometimes kidneys may shut down completely and a person may stop urinating while very ill and hospitalized. Then finally weeks or months later, when the acute illness has recovered, the kidneys may "wake back up" and restart filtration.

This is not without some lasting effects. After this injury, the kidneys often do not normalize to complete function. An episode of acute kidney injury or failure carries an increased risk of developing CKD. In fact, 31% of patients discharged from the hospital with a diagnosis of acute kidney injury develop CKD within one year (USRDS 2018 annual report). The dialysis treatment needed for a person with acute kidney failure is distinguishable from that needed for end-stage renal disease (ESRD). The former is recoverable and often temporary. This can be confusing for patients with ESRD on dialysis, as they may get a false sense of hope that their kidneys could recover as well.

So, are there any chronic kidney diseases that can recover? The short answer is yes. Some kidney diseases like lupus nephritis (lupus kidney disease) or certain types of glomerulonephritis can go into remission or even be cured with medications. However, CKD from diabetes or hypertension is typically not curable and rather, slowly progresses over the course of 10-20 years. The role of a nephrologist (kidney specialist) is to diagnose, treat kidney disease and to slow the progression of the kidney diseases we cannot cure. One of the mainstays of treatment is actually treating the underlying cause. For diabetes, this means strict glucose control with a goal hemoglobin A1c level less than 7%. Unfortunately, many patients are not referred to a nephrologist until late in the course of their disease, when there are less interventions available. This has a tremendous impact on both the person's care as well as the relationship between the kidney specialist and patient.

As a kidney specialist, it is challenging to meet a patient late in a disease course. The specialist must diagnose the patient and bring him/her to a level of acceptance regarding a terminal disease process, educate him about the disease and then also prepare him for a life-altering procedure. US data from 2011 reveal 42% of new dialysis starts had no prior nephrology care *(USRDS 2013 Annual Data Report: Table 1.f (Volume 2) Page 430 Analytical Methods)* despite studies showing better prognosis for patients when they are referred in early stages of kidney disease. Overall mortality and hospital length of stays are also higher in patients who had late referral to nephrologist *(AM J Med 2007, Outcomes in in patients with CKD referred late to a nephrologist)*. The national kidney foundation guidelines recommend referring patients to specialist kidney care services for any persons with progression of CKD or proteinuria (protein in urine). With increased public awareness about kidney disease and the treatment options, patients can be their own advocates in learning about CKD and specialty referral.

What are the stages of kidney disease? There are 5 progressive stages based on the severity of the decline in kidney function filtration or GFR (glomerular filtration rate).

- Stage 1 represents clinically undetectable kidney disease with a normal GFR but signs of kidney damage by urine testing (protein or blood in urine) or imaging.
- Stage 2 CKD represents a mild decline in GFR.
- Stage 3 is a moderate to a more severe decline in kidney function. This stage is the most prevalent.
- CKD stage 4 represents severe kidney dysfunction.
- Stage 5 represents a kidney reserve of under 15% and is the stage in which patients initiate dialysis.

A person with stage 5 chronic kidney disease on dialysis is said to have "end stage renal disease" (ESRD), the terminal point of the natural progression of CKD. Once a person is dialysis-dependent, the only way to restore health and stop dialysis is a kidney transplant.

What is dialysis? Dialysis is a way to remove toxins and fluid from the body when kidneys have failed. There are two forms of dialysis that patients can choose from: peritoneal (performed through the abdomen) and hemodialysis (through the blood). In 2016, there were over 700,000 persons with ESRD. Of persons newly starting on dialysis, 87% of individuals chose hemodialysis and 10% chose PD (*USRDS.org*). Hemodialysis can be performed either in a dialysis clinic or at home while peritoneal dialysis is solely self-administered by the patient at home.

Peritoneal dialysis (PD) is performed on a daily basis by the patient. The dialysis occurs through the body's own peritoneal membrane, a porous membrane filled with capillaries, which is like a cloth that covers the intestines and is used as the filter. Bags of fluid (dialysate) are instilled through a catheter tube surgically implanted into the abdominal cavity. This procedure can be done manually as "exchanges" during the day or automatically through a "cycler" machine at night while sleeping.

Hemodialysis (HD) is most commonly performed in a dialysis clinic and requires minimal work by the patient. The patient attends a dialysis treatment center 3 days a week for 4-hour sessions. The entire procedure is performed by a dialysis technician and the HD machine. HD requires access to the blood for filtration and is performed ideally through an arteriovenous (AV) fistula in the arm. This fistula is a surgical connection between the large artery and vein in the arm in order to create a high rate of blood flow. Two needles are placed in the fistula and attached to a dialysis machine, which removes blood on one side and then replaces the filtered or cleansed blood on the other side after cycling through the dialysis filter in the machine. Unfortunately, despite the superiority of an AV fistula as the choice for vascular access, most patients in the U.S. start HD with a temporary catheter placed in the large neck veins into the heart. The reasons for this are multifactorial but include in part late or lack of kidney specialist referrals as well as a lack of education of the patients regarding their disease and dialysis options.

As awareness and education increases, slowly more patients are choosing home dialysis. There are many clear benefits of home dialysis over in-center HD. These benefits include improved quality of life and energy levels, freedom to work or travel, less dietary restrictions, and less hospitalizations. Both the very young and old can be trained on home dialysis. The disproportionate use of in-center HD as the main treatment modality is multifactorial, but nephrologists must take responsibility for doing our part in fully educating and providing patients with their options. Patient quality of life and freedom are not often measured, but the importance of these factors cannot be overstated.

A bit about me. I am a nephrologist (kidney medical doctor). The pre-fix "neph" comes from the Greek word "nephrós" meaning kidney. I did not always know I wanted to be a kidney specialist. In medical school, my initial interest was in surgery after an exhilarating month on a transplant surgery rotation. I gained a profound respect and admiration for both surgery and organ transplantation watching these operations, lasting up to 8 hours long. The detailed work of the surgeon delicately dissecting the ureter from the donor then carefully sewing it into the recipient's bladder with great precision was like watching a work of art come to life. I appreciated the methodical nature of these operations.

While transplant surgery was exciting, meaningful work, I realized the field did not provide many opportunities for preventative work or disease management. I had a strong desire to do something for patients before they were at this terminal point. I valued the longevity of relationships with patients and the breadth of knowledge of different fields I would gain with Internal Medicine.

Internal Medicine physicians treat all of the body's systems and manage chronic diseases. They value preventative care and manage everything from diabetes and high blood pressure to shock and heart failure. After a 3-year residency in Internal Medicine, I felt I wanted an additional challenge in the medical field that would draw-on my love for solving problems and utilize my sharp critical thinking skills in formulating diagnoses. This search led me to explore a fellowship in the sub-specialty of Nephrology. In the medical community, Nephrologists are often known as the "nerds" of medicine. The reason being is that nephrology requires a deep understanding of pathophysiology in addition to a methodical and scientific approach to problem-solving. I like to think of it at times as detective work.

Each day, I feel as if I am piecing together a puzzle in working with diagnosis and treatment plans for patients with kidney disease. Each patient is unique, and thus I never tire of this problem-solving quest. Beyond the puzzle solving, I find the personal connections with my patients to be incredibly fulfilling. I work closely with these patients and their families over often many years. I witness their disease develop and how it affects their life, and their mental well-being. I enjoy the process of getting to know them as a whole person and building a trusting relationship. It truly is a privilege to have this role in their lives and find myself personally invested to improve or stabilize their condition. I recall several times cheering with the clinic nurse when a patient's labs resulted showing remission of his glomerulonephritis and another patient's acute kidney injury recovered and I was able to call him and let him know his past dialysis session was the very last one for him.

One of the most rewarding aspects of my work as a nephrologist is when a reversible cause is found. There is nothing more gratifying than "saving" someone from dialysis. I experienced one of those pivotal moments four years ago when I was consulted to see a patient, Mr. W, an African-American man with advanced prostate cancer. Mr. W was admitted to the hospital with acute kidney failure. The medical and urological team felt strongly that I start him on dialysis, but I believed that we could potentially circumvent dialysis if we treated the probable underlying obstruction causing the kidney failure instead. I asked Mr. W to put his trust in me – a complete stranger. Thankfully, he did. We put tubes in his kidneys to alleviate the blockages and his kidney failure gradually reversed. He has been in stable stage 3 CKD for nearly 3 years and went on to get his prostate cancer treated and in remission. Mr. W now goes hiking with his wife and travels around the country. These activities would have been almost impossible for him to do while on dialysis. Through experiences like these, I have learned that a diagnosis of CKD does not have to mean a diminished quality of life.

The unique thing about kidney disease is that most of the patients do not know they have it when they come for a consultation. Unprepared, they often look quizzically at me with skepticism, as if maybe I have the wrong person or chart. It's hard to blame one, as kidney disease is a silent disease. Also, many are unfamiliar with the disease because it does not get much publicity. We don't hear about CKD as often as heart disease or cancer. It affects 15 % of Americans (*USRDS.org 2018*) and one-third of adults with diabetes (CDC statistics). Yet, only 10 % of people with CKD are aware of their kidney disease (USRDS.org 2018). In fact, each year, it kills more people than breast or prostate cancer.

(*NIDDK, https://www.niddk.nih.gov/health-information/health-statistics/kidney-disease*).

During my medical training, and even in my career as a nephrologist, it has not been uncommon to hear other medical professionals make comments, such as "the heart is more important than the kidneys" or "It's fine, the patient can just go on dialysis if the kidneys fail." Post-operatively, when consulted to see a patient in kidney failure in the hospital, I am often limited in what I can do to help. Within the medical community, surgical needs and/or other vital organ systems are often a priority and it is not unusual for hospital staff to default to the surgeon or cardiologist and the kidneys to take a "backseat." The unfortunate truth is that the patient's failing kidneys are not uncommonly due to iatrogenic (healthcare-induced) causes such as blood loss anemia, low blood pressure, IV contrast dye for scans and interventional procedures, and nephrotoxic medications. The mindset has been difficult to change. The at-times flippant attitude toward dialysis as a modality for kidney failure dismisses the impact of kidney disease on patients' lives. Not only does the need for dialysis increase illness, hospitalizations, and mortality, it also has a tremendous impact on quality of life.

The other sad reality is that only half of patients who start dialysis will still be alive after 5 years. As a nephrologist I often must be the "bad guy"— the one who tells them what they cannot eat, cannot drink and cannot do. With such little time left, life's simple pleasures are taken away. Many patients struggle with feeling a loss of control, a decrease in quality of life, and depression. The depression and sometimes despair can be felt when I round in the dialysis unit. Many patients cannot bear to stay awake during their treatments and prefer to take medications to sleep through it. Others can be angry and irritable. I try to imagine what it feels like, being confined to a machine for 12 hours a week. Many patients often ask to shorten their treatment, skip sessions, or cheat on their diets. This short-term relief has long-term negative effects. The statistics show elevated phosphorous and potassium levels from dietary non-adherence and shortened or missed treatments ultimately increase morbidity and mortality, so these seemingly trivial choices can have serious consequences.

Patients always remember the nephrologist who started them on dialysis. Reasonably so, as often patients first meet their nephrologist in the hospital when they have a 5-10% kidney capacity and have reached a point where their body can no longer function. They are typically in stage 4 or 5 kidney disease and "crash" into dialysis for the first time in the hospital. During my fellowship, I was that nephrologist for many patients. I completed my fellowship in a hospital in Southern California that had a large population of underserved patients without access to regular healthcare. These patients were often admitted to the hospital in chronic renal failure, unbeknownst to them.

One particular woman I recall, Ms. S, a Latina in her 60s, was admitted to my hospital multiple times within a month or so with what is known as "uremia" or the clinical manifestations of renal failure. Her lungs had filled with fluid, her potassium and phosphorous were sky-high, and her blood was acidic. The signs were all chronic and "end stage" from years of diabetes. She stared at me in fear but adamantly shook her head "no" when I told her she needed to start dialysis. As I read her abnormal EKG, I became concerned she could suffer a cardiac arrhythmia and arrest at any moment. I pleaded with her in the ER and then later in the medical ward to start dialysis. The human body is amazing, and she "bounced" back and forth to the hospital three separate times before finally accepting that she had no other option but to start dialysis. While many patients in the United States, like Ms. S, may view dialysis as a scary, daunting form of treatment (perhaps, similar in many respects to the negative perceptions of chemotherapy treatment for cancer patients), many patients from outside the United States came to our hospital with suitcases straight from the airport, after flying miles from their country in a rush to get dialysis in the United States. Despite the drawbacks of dialysis, it is a life-saving procedure that does not exist in some countries or is reserved for an elite minority.

One of the most striking patients I started on dialysis, was a fellow physician. As a young attending physician, I was somewhat intimidated when I received the consult to go see "Dr. J," a well-known specialist at my hospital. I reviewed the chart in depth beforehand and upon interviewing him, quickly realized the probable diagnosis, end-stage renal failure from undiagnosed glomerulonephritis. I biopsied his kidney to confirm the diagnosis and went over the results. He had no symptoms and could not believe the diagnosis. He had been taking blood pressure medication but was not seeing a physician or having lab tests on a regular basis. Caring for his patients was his top priority. And as many physicians do, he neglected his own basic care. A simple blood and urine test would have led to a diagnosis and thus to treatment. I related to him in a way I had not before with other patients. The thought "this could have been me" popped into my head.

My medical career has given me the ability to be a fortune teller in a way. I deal with the "end stage" of a horrible disease. If I could change one thing about my work as a nephrologist, it would be to have the opportunity to see more patients when they are younger so I can tell them, "I see your future if this path continues," and counsel them on ways to protect their kidneys—an organ most people do not think about getting a "check-up" for.

I hope that one day I have fewer patients whom I meet for the first time at the doorstep of dialysis or ESRD. The only way this will be possible is if more people are aware of kidney disease—its causes, its prevalence, and how it can be detected.

This book is an incredible starting point for a national conversation on kidney disease. I am continuing this campaign through opening my own medical practice where I plan to hold seminars, classes and provide information online to the public. I am actively researching potential treatments for kidney disease and have a hope of a cure in the future. Through partnerships with community clinics, primary care providers and non-profit organizations like 1in9, we can all do our part to spread the word and educate the community. If you are reading this book, then I also welcome you to be part of the "kidney tribe!"

Elise Barney, DO is a board-certified nephrologist, internist, clinician educator and advocate for kidney disease awareness. Dr. Barney is an assistant professor of Medicine at Midwestern University and the University of Arizona College of Medicine and has been a Nephrology educator and preceptor at Banner University Medical Center. In addition, she presents Nephrology topics and research at state and national conferences. Dr. Barney is active in educating the public on kidney disease and dialysis. She is the founder of Mind Body Kidney, LLC, a unique medical practice offering personalized specialty care with a holistic view. Dr. Barney lives in Phoenix, AZ and enjoys traveling, photography, hiking and fitness in her free time.

Helping Patients Thrive at Home

Dr. Sachin Desai

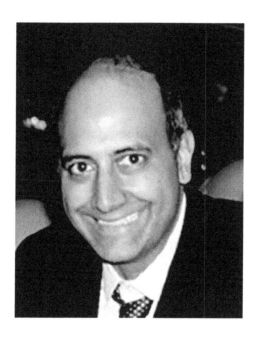

The astonishing fact that 1 in 9 Americans has chronic kidney disease may come as a surprise to patients when they are first diagnosed with this disease. It may be best to think of kidney disease as a continuum to decrease anxiety associated with the diagnosis. It is not until the later stages of kidney disease when preparations must be made for renal replacement therapies. Education regarding what do when faced with the ultimate decision is key to coping with kidney failure.

When faced with the prospect of kidney failure, patients have few choices. Renal replacement therapy choices include peritoneal dialysis, hemodialysis, and transplant. If appropriate, patients may also opt to choose palliative care options should they decide on not doing dialysis. The latter option which includes hospice is a deeply personal decision which will not be the focus of this section.

Kidney failure manifests itself silently in most cases until it is too late. Since only laboratory tests identify kidney disease at early stages, seeking routine care from a health professional is essential. Preventive care discussed earlier in this book is critical in slowing the progression of chronic kidney disease. It is not until later stages of kidney disease, typically stage 3 and higher, when patients are referred to a nephrologist.

Common symptoms of kidney failure include leg swelling, shortness of breath, fatigue, nausea, poor appetite, and itching. As many of these symptoms are nonspecific, laboratory tests are used to diagnose kidney failure.

In the United States, greater than 90% of patients do In-center hemodialysis. In-center hemodialysis is a modality in which patients do dialysis three times per week at a dialysis center on average 3-4 hours depending on the individual. Patients many times feel wiped out after dialysis with recovery times varying. Longer treatment times may help alleviate some of the symptoms. Nocturnal dialysis where treatments are run at night for 6-8 hours may be an alternative for certain patients.

Dialysis can also be done at home using two methods: Peritoneal dialysis and home hemodialysis. Dialysis at home is done in a comfortable setting. The treatments are done more frequently, closer mimicking the natural physiology of the kidney. Many side effects patient may have with in-center hemodialysis are alleviated by the increased frequency of dialysis. Patients generally have fewer complaints of fatigue, cramping, and swelling.

Peritoneal dialysis uses the natural membrane of the abdominal wall as a filter to remove toxins from the body along with the extra fluid. A tube is surgically inserted into the abdomen. Dialysate fluid is put into the abdomen (referred to as peritoneal space) via a surgically inserted tube. The fluid dwells in the body for a specified amount of time before it is exchanged for new dialysate fluid. Exchanges can be done manually every 6 to 8 hours depending on the prescription or using a cycler which automates the process and is done nightly, while the patient sleeps.

Home hemodialysis is most commonly done as a short daily therapy done 5-6 times per week. The prescription can be modified for longer dialysis runs done 4-5 times per week. Short daily therapy allows patients to dialyze in their own home on their own schedule. Patients thus can keep an active lifestyle.

A preemptive transplant is an underutilized option. Preemptive transplant is defined as kidney transplantation from a living or deceased donor before the kidneys failing to the point dialysis is needed. To pursue this option, one must be under the care of a nephrologist and be referred to a transplant center earlier in the CKD process. Many transplant centers will start work-up for preemptive transplantation when a patient's glomerular filtration rate (GFR) is less than 20 ml/min.

It is unfortunate, many patients are not aware of the different options available to them for dialysis. Many organizations such as 1in9 are helping raise awareness so patients can choose the option which best suits them. As a practicing nephrologist with the country's largest nephrology group, my partners and I have a robust education program available to our patients. In other geographic regions, there may be limited resources. Other times when being diagnosed with acute kidney failure, the quickest option in clearing toxins from a patient may be hemodialysis. The patient, overwhelmed with the new diagnosis, may not process the different options available. The medical community must do a better job circling back with patients after starting in-center dialysis to focus on the other options.

Each of the options presented thus far have advantages and disadvantages. Surveys amongst nephrologists have shown a preference of home dialysis should he or she develop kidney failure. In reality, less than 10% of patients are choosing this route, however. My personal bias lies towards short daily hemodialysis with NxStage, although peritoneal dialysis would be a close second choice. Having worked with the patient over the last 5 years building one of the larger home hemodialysis clinics in the Southwest, I have been amazed by how well my patients have thrived. Patients are happy and able to live their lives in full when dialyzing at home. The greatest differences I have seen are a decreased number of hospitalizations and increased energy levels.

Much of what I presented thus far is background, without discussing personal experiences. A story however is not complete without sharing specific patient experiences. Given federal regulations which prevent the use of patient identifiers, I will speak in more general terms. My patients who are using NxStage short daily home hemodialysis are motivated. They want to feel better and have embraced the challenge of beating kidney disease. They have sought out alternatives to in-center dialysis to live a fuller life.

An illustrative example is a young gentleman who had trouble maintaining normal blood pressures on dialysis despite medication. He would have leg cramping with dialysis. Fluid could not be removed as blood pressures dropped too low. He had already failed a transplant and has been waiting indefinitely for another transplant due to his high immune sensitivity. After much deliberation, he chose to give NxStage a try. Within a month, he noticed he was not as wiped out after dialysis. The extra energy kickstarted his desire to work. He changed professions and now teaches firearm training to law enforcement officials. NxStage offered him the flexibility to dialyze around his schedule. He no longer is wiped out for hours after dialysis. In fact, the energy level has increased to the point where he is thinking about not getting a kidney transplant.

Another patient, a father of a young boy, transplanted kidney failed after a few years. He had been doing in-center hemodialysis before discovering NxStage. Before home hemodialysis, he had symptoms of low energy and difficulty managing electrolytes. Using NxStage, he found through short daily dialysis five times per week; he felt better. He has become more engaged in his young son's life feeling well enough to take trips to Disneyland or the beach. Additionally, he is pursuing higher education within his profession.

A young female patient was doing in-center dialysis and frequently missed dialysis. Her rural clinic would not accept her as a patient for home dialysis due to history non-compliance with dialysis. Through a compassionate team approach and behavioral contract, the patient was started on NxStage at my clinic. Through NxStage, she was able to stay home post-pregnancy, taking care of her premature baby who is now thriving.

These are only a few examples of how NxStage home hemodialysis has impacted the quality of life positively.

The gold standard treatment for renal failure is a kidney transplant. However, many patients, unfortunately, are not candidates. Due to the shortage of organs available for transplantation, wait times can be 5+ years. Newer advances in transplant medicine have the potential to lead to a larger number of patients being a match and less patient rejecting transplanted organs.

The future for patients with kidney disease is bright. In 2011, the Food and Drug Administration created an "Innovation Pathway" to shorten the time and cost it takes to develop, assess and review medical devices. The pilot program was meant to fast-track treatments for the patients who need it most, in this case, end-stage kidney disease patients. New technologies from compact home dialysis machines to wearable kidney devices are on the horizon. Miniaturization of existing devices with nanotechnology will one day lead to implantable artificial kidneys. The potential use of regenerative medicine through stem cells is actively being researched and breakthroughs could lead to avoiding dialysis altogether.

Sachin Desai, MD is a practicing Board Certified nephrologist passionate about home dialysis. He is a partner at Arizona Kidney Disease and Hypertension Center. Dr. Desai serves as medical director for several dialysis clinics in Phoenix, AZ. He is Chairman of Medicine at HonorHealth Deer Valley Medical Campus. He is among a select group of nephrologists to sit on the Fresenius Joint Venture Council. Dr. Desai has developed one of the largest NxStage home hemodialysis clinics in the western United States in collaboration with Fresenius Medical Care. He is a strong advocate for home dialysis. Dr. Desai has been Raymond Scott's nephrologist for the over 5 years.

Bank on Me

Dr. Jean Robey

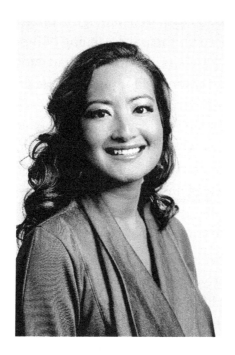

I was the second opinion. Unfortunately, laboratory numbers do not waiver in an office air-conditioned breeze or erase in the sand against the waves of the day or the persuasion of the wanting that comes to sit in a 10 feet x 10 feet room to find out a second or third or fourth opinion.

The science unfolded as I leafed through the pages and asked questions. He availed himself and his posture said he feared the worst. "Tell it to me straight," his shoulders braced, and his facial muscles tensed. He did not trust me, but he did not have to yet.

"Well, the labs show your kidney function is quite impaired and of course your blood pressure is both a cause and a consequence," I maintained the first opinion.

The decision to biopsy the kidney for a diagnosis had already been made by another twice and the biopsies laid bare the findings of a genetic disease and acquired damage in progressive decline. The word "fibrosis" glared on the pages, telling of function permanently lost. He was only 32 years old and he had Alport syndrome and hypertension related chronic kidney disease. He presented physically fit and as often the case the numbers did not describe him fully. I saw in his eyes a kind of yield and fear and he folded his hands into his lap with the finality of an accepted vulnerability as I carefully told him what he already had heard and a little more about why he needed to listen this time. He was unsure if he was supposed to be hopeful or hopeless. Humans are not fashioned for chronic illness when we are young. When we are young, we are invincible.

"You are not invincible," I cut directly at the root of the budding conflict, "but you are not without hope," I pruned further. "You have to try to see the full forest for the trees and practice a kind of multi approach to a problem. We will do what we can to protect what kidney function you have left AND we will also prepare you for what comes next as it is indeed coming. My hope is to have you transplanted before ever needing dialysis. It is a tight window but that is where we can hope to be crafty and timely."

It is something to have a doctor tell you your kidneys are failing with certainty. I could feel the weight of the seriousness fall like a gavel onto a young man's life line.

"When do I need dialysis exactly?" he worried.

Exact is a notion of control and the use of the word "exactly" is the spiraling out of control of a person. Kidney disease has so few avenues for control in the way we scrap to find it.

"The need for dialysis is up for negotiation. The labs tell me some part of the picture and clues for a course and YOU tell me the rest. The young and otherwise healthy can tolerate so much more than the older or ill," I revealed and made him accountable for his part of the journey forward.

"I don't feel so young," he cowered and laughed.

"Trust me, you are very young still," I assured.

His youth became our ally. His engagement the thread to which I began to sew a hopefully seamless stitch to bridge the unknown to all he knew thus. We spent that first day affirming what he already had been told but, in that revisit, and in the respectful request to have him trust me as I designed his best paths, he agreed to stop seeking opinions but to start the larger work of accepting the eventuality of a different life than which he fathomed altogether.

"You will need to trust me now," I asked, and he met me 85% of the way, leaving a little window to escape from.

Months went by, and we busied ourselves laboratory analysis and renegotiations. His numbers climbed and he began to grow weaker and fatigued easily.

"It's hard for me to tell the guys at work I'm tired or that I'm sick. I don't look sick, but I feel so tired often," he confessed. He was a Staff Sergeant already decorate beyond the usual limits with 4 commendations and 1 achievement after 8 years of waking at 5 AM to serve. I wrote letters to support his justified decrease in stamina as his kidney function dropped well below 15%.

To whom it may concern:

Please be considerate of Mr. Banks failing health. He is still able to work, but you will find him unable to excel as he used to. He is in the process of waiting for a kidney transplant and may be on dialysis soon.

Regards,

Dr. Jean Robey

Months went by, and he busied himself still living. Kidney failure did not need him to stop living. He worked and went to the gym. He dated and one day came with joyful news against the backdrop of kidney disease.

"I got married," he beamed. She was a lovely lady with rich brown hair and a kind of compassion in her that said she cared about his well-being and took him as he was and might become. Her children enter the marriage with his full interest. "I'm also now a father!" he prided.

Months went by, and he busied himself searching for alternatives where none truly existed.

"Can you tell me if Bardoxolone Methyl can help me? Can you request the drug company investigating it release it to me for compassionate use?" he phoned.

We discussed the reality of true change in his trajectory. "Stave the path," I convinced him, and the compassion hung in the air like the shadow of a noose. "It will not help you," I had to confess.

"Thank you for helping me to consider it and to understand why not," he acquiesced though I could hear the neck of hope break under pressure to be well again.

Simultaneously we sought out transplant listing, and he qualified easily being thankfully young and otherwise fit. Waiting active on the list though left an uncertain future but a future with notions of feeling well again.

"It is not a cure but a treatment. It represents for you the best course forward though," I explained. We kept the champagne chilled.

Too many months went by, and he fell a victim of depression and self-doubt. The marriage was troubled by the strain of unexplainable trials. I knew he was less the man he wanted and less the man she married, but I wanted them to hold on as a transplant could mean so much more to enjoy.

"I can't do the things we fell in love doing together," he admitted, and his voice yearning pushed on my heart. "We used to hike and go to the gym and I just can't," he acknowledged painfully.

"Hold on friend," I tried to bolster him. We addressed anxiety and depression, and he thanked me for the measure of thought to do so. Kidney failure lays in the back waiting for all organs to fail around it and effect it is including the breaking of the heart and the crushing of the soul.

"You are only human to be uncertain and diminished by uncertainty but think no more of that. You will be ok if you can weather better this time for just a time longer," I swore. So, the stigma of antidepressants was negated, and we embraced aid.

More months went by, and with the rise of his numbers that herald the growing dominance of kidney failure, he began to return every four weeks. Each lab draw harked the office to "check on him."

"Hello?" he would answer the phone.

"Hello, Mr. Banks, it's Dr. Robey's assistant. Are you feeling ok?" the medical assistant would inquire. His numbers increased steadily, and he flirted with high potassium and acidosis. The numbers told part of a story. He needed to tell the rest as agreed upon that first day.

"Should I feel badly?" he worried, "I'm just tired," he offered.

"As tired as last month or more so?" the medical assistant would delve.

"Same as last month," he would confirm. The relief of no new symptoms and his stability on the edge, nervously bought another four weeks at a time

The careful diet revisited, the appointment to come where a doctor could examine and review reminded, the disconnected call, and the man standing on the precipice of the unknown waiting all played over and over each month. I caught him falling in doubt each month.

"I'm sorry we must perhaps frighten you each month by calling to triage you," I explained in the office. The emotional fatigue as heavy as the physical told me he needed some perspective. "It is the only way we can ascertain if you are decompensating and that we must switch gears. I know it is hard to know if you are to answer a certain way. I know it is a constant worry if something sudden will happen in the middle of the night. It is not this way with you in your youth. We will see something coming. We call to understand better the laboratory numbers not to tell you bad news."

He thanked us for our concern and booked the next round of labs and appointment.

Months went by, and he relaxed under the scrutiny and interrogations. He learned just to answer the call, "Nope, I'm the same. Just tired. Thanks!"

Months went by, and he researched the various forms of dialysis, and he felt confident he would be capable of self-care. He chose to consider peritoneal dialysis, and I was excited he was growing confident enough to engage and command his chronic illness instead of letting it drown him in lost plans and perceived halvings of a man's self-worth. "I think I can do this," he couraged.

"I know you can," I attested.

Months became the measure of our relationship and the substance of familiarity until it was years.

Finally, one October afternoon he came to my office. The day was ordinary and the weather not yet cool in Arizona. He was stable and his mood level. He was unchanged and frozen in his stance while I examined him. Suddenly I was looking over his shoulder listening to his heart sounds when I saw in the window a bird fly by. In my soul, I felt a sadness and loss of a kind, but quickly it displaced with a reason. A clear wave washed over the sands of the day, and there lingered a thought, "He will not be back in my office the way he is today." That person would disappear. That "him" was here to say goodbye. He would be in the time I would see him next transformed. It was not a sad dismissal but a welcoming soon of a new version of a man.

"Michael," I said taking the earpieces of my stethoscope out. "I have a thought, and I need to tell you. I need just to see if it comes to fruition. I suddenly felt like I will not see you again in this office quite the same."

He cringed a bit to wonder what that ominous statement meant.

"I mean," I relieved, "I think you will get a kidney transplant before our next appointment! Moreover, I think this part of our journey is completing."

He laughed perplexed and unsure of such a bold statement. I laughed too at such a prophecy and the power to make it but made him promised he would call me second or third to please confirm this feeling I could not deny. "Please do call me! I am certain you will get a transplant," I smiled convinced.

"Sure, Dr. Robey," he humored. "I'll call you," he rolled his mind's eyes and left laughing.

Nearly a month passed.

"Dr. Robey," my medical assistant called out to me as she entered my office. My head was down buried in pages of papers to address and forms to sign.

"Yes," I answered, not making eye contact.

"This message was left for you on the portal," my medical assistant slid in front of my face to register.

"Please let Dr. Robey know at your earliest convenience, I am at Mayo clinic and received a kidney from a deceased donor. I got the call on Thanksgiving! I'm in the Phoenix Mayo and doing well. Thank you, Dr. Robey, you saved my life, I would have never made it without you. I can't thank you and your staff enough for all of your support in getting me here and keeping me on track." - Mike

I am sure no commendation has hung so heavy on a man as the thanks a healthy, prosperous patient does on a doctor. I can find no better achievement in my profession. That window Mr. Michael Banks left open to escape from on the first day became not as enticing as the door we opened together for him to leave and venture down into a wide, long hallway of living.

We are all on a journey of many paths and understanding our potential, actualizing our manifest destiny, and surviving our given tribulations is the purpose of living. We are looking for answers, aids, choices, preparation, hope, guidance, and time used wisely. We are 1 in 9 with kidney disease. We hope that someone champions us and takes us to the next level and then the next level and on and on and finds us any new or current possibility. We look for hope. We look for coping. We need attention. "We" could be YOU. You could be 1 in 9.

Have you found the sound of your drum?

Jean Robey MD is a practicing Nephrologist in Arizona. She is an enthusiastic educator and supporter of patients and families and aspiring young adults. She is a writer and poet. She is deeply in love with her profession and the opportunities that are made to meet people where they stand and help them get to where they are destined in great form and with great company. She is among all things an excited mother, a happy wife, a grateful daughter, a proud sibling, and a humbled contributor who thanks readers for taking their time to read her offerings. "We stand to only make a small counter measure in our lifetime. Let us stand to do if just that." - Jean Robey MD

I Am Not My Disease

Raymond Scott

Over the twenty-one years as an end-stage renal disease patient, I have had many doctors, of all types. From Dr. Mishler to Dr. Desai, and all of the other Nephrologists and their teams in between from AKDHC that have cared for me since my kidneys first failed, to my Cardiology team, VA doctors, and so many others - I've been very fortunate to receive exceptional care.

My wife Analyn and I have always been vocal and active participants in all aspects of my health with my medical care teams, which I believe is a crucial factor in my longevity. It's my responsibility to take charge of my health, but I also need to know that my voice is heard and feel confident in those whom I am entrusting my health and life to.

To stress the importance of being your own biggest advocate, I would like to highlight two very memorable, yet completely different experiences that I had recently. Both took place last year with two different medical professionals that were meeting me for the first time.

The first experience was with a Urologist. Earlier last year I had some health challenges that we were trying to figure out. A CT scan was performed and showed that I had multiple cysts on my kidneys, a few that were questionable, so it was recommended that I consult with a Urologist.

You may be wondering why a Urologist when I haven't been able to urinate for years, I did too at first. I learned that Urologists focus on anatomical disorders of the kidneys and urinary tract, treat kidney problems including blockages and kidney cancer, and can perform surgeries if necessary.

Analyn and I pulled up my report from a CT scan done a year or so earlier to bring to my appointment for comparison and were shocked to see "polycystic kidney disease" listed in a section of the report that we didn't notice before. Keep in mind; this was the first time that we had ever seen "polycystic kidney disease" in any of my records. Knowing that this is a hereditary disease we were concerned about our own children. We did some research and were surprised but somewhat relieved to learn that 90% of people on dialysis for eight years or more develop "acquired cystic kidney disease," which is not hereditary. We believed that was likely the case for me but wanted to make sure.

Now we had even more questions, and wanting to be fully prepared, we took the time to order the DVD's from my last three CT scans along with the full reports to bring to our first consultation for the Urologist to review. In addition to these two most recent scans, we also obtained one that was done about seven years earlier. The latest CT scan had also been sent before my appointment for his review.

We sat in the freezing exam room waiting for the doctor to enter, with the reports and discs in hand. The appointment started like most did when meeting with a new specialist, but it ended very differently than we expected. We explained how we stumbled on the report listing "polycystic kidney disease" and our concerns around it because of our children, and of course, wanting to know the status of the cysts that brought us to him. We explained how we gathered the reports and discs for the three scans and how we thought they would help tell a story. He refused to take and review them, instead, telling us to take those to our nephrologist to answer our "polycystic kidney" questions.

He explained that his only concern was the cysts, that he needed to order another CT scan with contrast dye to give him a better view to determine if it was cancer or not. We were not prepared for what he said next, "if it is cancer I need to determine if you're even healthy enough for surgery because you've been on dialysis for so long. We will need to way out the risk of surgery versus your life expectancy on dialysis." As we were left dumbfounded, he tried to reassure us of his experience and skill level, that I was in good hands, and to focus on getting the scan for him to review and go from there. I felt invisible.

I remember leaving the appointment pissed off, telling Analyn, "he only saw my disease, he did not see me!" In all my years of fighting this battle, that was the first time I truly felt like I was being treated like a number, not the determined, strong man who continued to beat the odds and who was full of life that stood before him.

I moved forward with the scan and was grateful that it confirmed that I did not have cancer, then transferred my care to another Urologist that could "see" me.

The second experience couldn't be further from the first. At my annual exam with my VA Primary Care doctor, he advised that as a 50-year-old African-American male I was due for a colonoscopy and submitted the request for a consult.

The day of my consult with the Gastroenterologist at the VA I was expecting to be taken into a standard examination room, but instead was walked directly into her office. There were pictures of her family on her desk, and she had my medical history pulled up on her computer screen to go over with us. She was amazed at how good I looked for all that I had been through. As we discussed my history, she combed through the information with intrigue and awe. She paused for a moment, looked at me and said, "When the consult came through, and I saw your medical history, I wanted to meet you in person and take the time to assess your current health to determine if and when we should proceed with a colonoscopy." She paused again, then said, "I'm fighting back the tears because when I saw your history, I was fully expecting you to be wheeled into my office in a wheelchair, but instead I saw this young, vibrant, healthy-looking man walk in."

She wanted to give my body a rest from a recent procedure I had but deemed me healthy for a colonoscopy to be scheduled a few months later. Not only did her outlook and this experience clearly brighten her day, but it did mine as well…I was truly seen.

PART 6:

The Drumbeat for Regenerative Medicine

The Future is NOW!

Analyn Scott

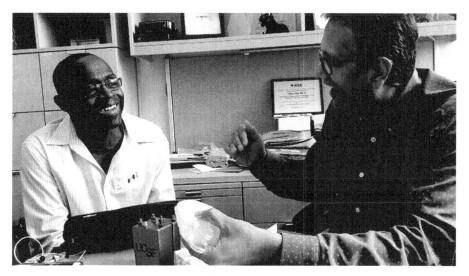

Raymond Scott and Shuvo Roy, Ph.D., USCF

What started as a typical monthly Nephrology appointment for Raymond created a spark of curiosity that ignited my belief that Regenerative Medicine holds the answers to a cure for kidney disease and ESRD.

I'm not sure how many months into Raymond's home hemodialysis journey we were in, but I recall us marveling at how great Raymond's lab results were and how great he was feeling compared to in-center dialysis. This modality gave us much hope for a longer future, especially since Raymond wasn't eligible for another transplant, but I still posed the question to Dr. Desai as to whether or not Raymond was on the best modality, and what options may be coming up in the future. He confirmed that for now, Raymond was on the best modality for him, but there was some innovative research being conducted in the field of regenerative medicine and bio-engineering that could be promising. Hearing about research around a wearable kidney or implantable bio-artificial kidney was very intriguing and exciting.

When I got home, I started to do more research. Google and YouTube were my friends as I followed one clue to another and so on. That's when I stumbled across TED talks from 2009 and 2011 that Dr. Anthony Atala from Wake Forest had given. He shared how he was able to use a patient's own stem cells and a 3-D printer to create a bladder that he was successfully able to implant into a young man... without the need of anti-rejection medications! There was great hope that the same could be done for kidneys, but we were at least a decade out since kidneys are much more complex.

From that moment forward I established my belief that a solution would be developed that would allow Raymond, and millions of others, to have a functioning kidney(s) without the need for anti-rejection medication. Therefore, when we founded 1in9, it made perfect sense to have Awareness, Prevention, and Regenerative Medicine as our 3 key pillars.

We have had the privilege to connect and, in some cases, collaborate with some of the absolute best in the field of Nephrology, Regenerative Medicine and their respective fields of medicine, and Engineering.

Dr. Zain Khalpey's bio is beyond impressive, but the man himself even more so. As a world-renowned Cardiothoracic surgeon with experience and a focus in areas such as heart transplantation, artificial heart programs, cell & molecular medicine and regenerative medicine, we were honored and extremely grateful for Dr. Khalpey to become a member of 1in9's Medical Advisory Board. Being all too familiar with the direct connection between heart disease & kidney disease, Dr. Khalpey brings an incredible amount of knowledge and experience that will benefit 1in9.

We are equally honored and thrilled to collaborate with the University of Arizona's Division of Nephrology Chief Prabir Roy-Chaudhury, MD, PhD. Raymond and I serve on the patient advisory Council that he established, and we are grateful to have Dr. Roy-Chaudhury on our 1in9 Medical Advisory Board. His passion to understand and promote the needs of CKD and ESRD patients has been a breath of fresh air.

Dr. Roy Chaudhury is also a national co-chair of the Kidney Health Initiative - a public-private partnership between the American Society of Nephrology and U.S. Food and Drug Administration to develop and bring therapies and devices to CKD patients more quickly. During one of our first meetings down in Tucson, he shared an analogy that really stood out to me, especially given my background in Information Technology. A slide projected on the screen showed an image of IBM mainframe computers filling up a room next to an image of a smartphone, explaining how much of the computing that used to take the resources of all those mainframe computers could now be done on a smartphone. The next slide showed pictures of the early dialysis machines from over 40 years ago next to images of dialysis machines used in most dialysis clinics and hospitals today. Both were similar in size without much change. With all of the technological advancements in so many other areas, why haven't we seen more done for dialysis and kidney disease? He proceeded to share disappointing disparities between funding allocated for kidney disease research compared to dollars being spent on research for cancer and many other diseases, that would help to provide at least a partial answer to the question and validate the accuracy of his analogy.

On one of our trips to Utah we scheduled a stop at BYU, where we had the opportunity to meet with chemical engineering professor Alonzo Cook, tour his lab, and learn much more about the background of tissue engineering, stem cells, and research taking place in his lab and around the world that will lead to breakthroughs to solve the global organ shortage.

During our RV tours in 2017, we were fortunate to meet and interview Dr. Giuseppe Orlando, Assistant Professor, Surgical Sciences - Transplant at Wake Forest, who has written a book and multiple research papers around such topics as state-of-the-art kidney transplantation, regenerative medicine and tissue engineering.

Our entire family was able to tour Dr. Benjamin D. Humphreys lab at Washington University in St. Louis. According to *humphreyslab.com*; "In the Humphreys Lab we are developing new and innovative treatments to help patients with kidney disease. We are using human stem cells to generate kidney organoids in a dish, with a goal of one day transplanting them into patients with kidney failure. We also study the kidney's ability to regenerate itself so that we can harness this ability for therapeutic uses."

It was absolutely fascinating for all of us to see the kidney organoids under the microscope. Although too small for use in humans now, Dr. Humphreys and his team are committed to continue working diligently on this and other research to bring about a cure for kidney disease.

That summer we went to the University of California, San Francisco (UCSF) to meet with Shuvo Roy, PhD, bioengineer, professor, and Technical Director and lead of The Kidney Project. Shuvo and his team are hard at work to create a bioartificial kidney as a permanent solution to end stage renal disease (ESRD).

On the table was an earlier prototype model next to the newer prototype of the bioartificial kidney that had been printed with a 3D printer. I'm sure you can imagine the feelings of hope and excitement Raymond and I both felt when we held the device in our hands. I could tell that our reaction was one that Shuvo Roy must see frequently, one that brought him joy, and I trust will continue to fuel his passion and determination to succeed in bringing this solution to the world.

Although we didn't get the opportunity to meet with William Fissell, MD on our east coast tour and stop at Vanderbilt University Medical Center, it's important to note that he is the Medical Director of the Kidney Project. I was very pleased to see the collaboration taking place on many levels. For Dr. Fissell to bring his medical and biological expertise, and to hear Shuvo Roy describe how his engineering mind was able to envision a revolutionary solution to dialysis and a permanent solution to end stage renal disease, sounded like a perfect match to me! Also, to see them work together from two different Universities and then also expand their collaboration efforts and include additional team members with the right skill sets needed from across the country was encouraging.

The Kidney Project has been conducting clinical safety trials, with the goal to be able to begin human trials in 2019. To learn more and stay informed I would recommend that you like and follow them on Facebook: The Kidney Project.

It's been so refreshing to see the passion and drive that each of these individuals mentioned has demonstrated to improve and save the lives of people with kidney disease. Each of them expressed an authentic desire for a cure for kidney disease to be developed and made available, even if someone else does it first.

PART 7:

The Wheels of Change

Dialysis and Me

Maryjane Hamilton

My mother, Eleanor, or El, as most called her, knew things. Knew things about life and having Fun. Knew things about kids. Knew how to talk to and have fun with kids. Knew how to still be a kid. She knew about adults and how to surprise and make them laugh. She knew how to be alone. She knew how to respect people. She embraced curiosity, and intrigue. She knew some secrets of New York City and its ghosts of the past. She knew the pleasures of people and she knew the feeling of being in love. She also knew how to do things. Things like: ice skate, roller skate, swim, body surf, jump waves, catch and cook crabs, kick a football higher than a large oak tree, plan a party, play cards, drink beer, sing for the fun of singing, dress up for Halloween and sometimes get into mischief.

She knew how to do things like, talk to strangers, taste weird food, laugh out loud, braid hair, ride roller coasters, ride Ferris wheels, kiss in the fun house, Christmas shop in secret, ride motorcycles, dive off the high dives, fearlessly. She knew how to be supportive, have neighborhood kids over to swim in summer, serve snacks and drinks, do housework all the while making it look fun and carefree with a smile. She could also do things like wear only red lipstick, match her outfit with black penny loafer shoes and dime store sunglasses and still look like a million dollars. She encircled the world with her ease of life and love of her family and friends.

This is a story about Eleanor and the man and love of her life, Lou, and the times in their life.

Let me now pull back the veil of so many years to recall past events of life before, during and after my experience with dialysis. So many emotions and feelings arise with the ghost of dialysis past. My mother, Eleanor Hamilton, was the person in my life who was afflicted with kidney failure, however it bled over to everyone associated in her life then and now, 45 years later. This is my perspective with early background life experiences, then the story that took me into the world of Kidney failure, dialysis, transplantation, invention, patents and adventure all blended with education, fun and sorrow beginning in the approximate year of 1970 when I was 15.

That was the year when I first heard and actually understood words such as a semipermeable membrane, osmosis, greater concentration, a lesser concentration of molecules and blood cleansing via a process called Dialysis. Applying the principles of dialysis for sustaining a person with Renal failure was called Hemodialysis, and "hooking up" to a machine to preserve or sustain a person's life. If there were no treatments, I was told, patients needing hemodialysis would "drown in their own fluids". More bluntly stated, die because our kidneys, unlike tonsils, are very necessary to continue life. Of course, I said I understood, but really was still a bit clouded by this whole "machine" thing and survival of someone I loved. A simple fix someone well-meaning said, and I was reassured the procedure was easy and safe. A quick attachment to a kidney machine and Voila! Blood cleaned, health regained! I had never heard of this, but good that there is such a "machine" I thought.

I had always been very squeamish about blood and bleeding so apprehension the first time I viewed my mother attached to the kidney machine was to be expected. The so-called quick fix and normal life that people mentioned seemed very distant when I entered the hospital dialysis ward that first day. There were about 8 patients in beds lined up against a wall with the 8 machines next to them. All of these a tangle of tubing, red tubing. The amount of blood I viewed that day, oh my! The day left me feeling weak and not knowing what the future for me would look like as my fear mounted each time the alarms on the machines beeped out their high-pitched squeals. My knees even buckled under me a couple of times trying to help dad steady my mom as we left the hospital.

My mom. A Fun-loving person with a lot of energy, kind, outgoing, considerate and often obstinate being tied as the youngest child with her twin brother in a family of 11 siblings, the majority being rowdy German brothers. Eleanor, growing up as the youngest girl, as you can imagine, was the sweetheart of all of her siblings, especially Butch, her twin. Her dad passed when she was a child and her mom was left without much support or means of support. She was undernourished and very thin when she met my dad, but happy and considerably carefree. They married in 1949, when she was 20 and dad 22. Mom and Dad were very close and loving, but Eleanor was a tenacious free-spirit. Dad was more reserved, and the match was a perfect contrast. My older brother, Lou Jr. and I seldom saw a cross look between mom and dad. We experienced love.

Lou, my dad, was a successful businessman, working many long hours in his self-started Lawn and Garden business during the peak season, and a devoted family man. Lou was so devoted to spending time together and traveling that my parents, brother and I were all in Disneyland the year it opened, 1955, however, I was just an infant. Crazy kids, those two, Lou and El were driving in a car about 2800 miles from NJ to CA with a 4-year-old and an infant on Route 66, the main highway cross country! Travel was a way of life whenever work would permit Lou to get away and due to the nature of his Lawn and Garden business in Northern NJ, the store was seasonal, and he had downtime from Thanksgiving to Easter. Road trips were their passion, as Lou and El enjoyed seeing as much of the U.S. as possible up close and personal and meeting its people in their own unique environment of hometown America.

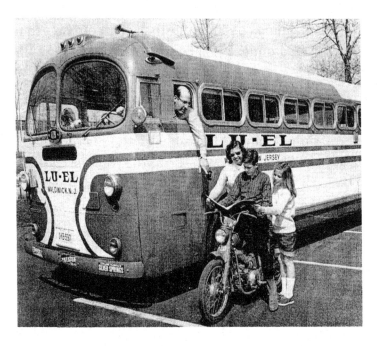

When we traveled Lou always had a loose plan for our journey in place, but the back roads and side adventures took us to many little places, museums, parks, stores, natural vistas, lakes, swimming pools, fishing docks, local tours, factory tours and wildlife not on the planned agenda. It was easy, down the road we went in a converted Bus, a 1940's Aerocoach.

This home on wheels was our life. They had tried other forms of travel, the usual hotels and travel trailers towed behind a car, but in about 1964 Lou began working on his first bus conversion and finished it quickly. He sold that first conversion, a school bus, immediately after completing it only after making a couple of trips with it. He then bought the Aerocoach with a motor and structure more suited to cross country travel. This remained the bus our whole family together traveled in the most. I do not know how many miles we logged on that bus during the years we crisscrossed throughout the southern and northern United States as well as some destinations in Canada, but we used it for many years. Sneaking away on weekend excursions into New England, Pennsylvania, visiting the rural regions of New Jersey, New York state, going to car races, Delaware, crabbing in Maryland and to Washington DC. We parked the bus right on the Mall in front of the Capitol in DC and mom cooked us dinner while we rode our bikes on the concrete apron around the Capitol building. This was a usual occurrence in many notable cities as people were not accustomed to seeing a privately-owned bus used for travel with sleeping and cooking accommodations and they extended a welcome with fascinated pleasure. Even the police were genuinely intrigued and supportive! We met interested and curious people with helpful attitudes and an eagerness to share secrets about their hometown. Dad was always eager as well to follow up on their recommendations and mom never knew a stranger! Dad had also added two small Honda motorcycles to the bus, one on the front and one on the back. Mom drove one and dad the other. I rode with dad, my brother with mom. This allowed us to really explore the back roads with intimacy. Many friendships were formed across the miles.

    Lou and El were quite a team. Mom even came up with a weird and unique collection of sorts that pretty much forced dad to stop in EVERY town and city we passed through. She collected pictures of Post Offices! Lou would have to park the bus, or motorcycle, get his 35 mm camera and take a picture of Eleanor standing in front of the post office, always wearing her sunglasses and her big smile. There are at least three thick photo albums of these vintage photos preserved, and my brother, Lou Jr., and I are in many of them with mom. It was travel at a snail's pace with her hobby, but we loved it. Dad would stop and turn around for us kids too if we saw something that interested us, and that was usually a candy store or a swimming pool.

Lou had been raised in New Jersey and had a natural propensity for all things mechanical. He attended school only until the eighth grade and dropped out. This was partly due to his poor grades in some academic classes but also because the school teachers and other school personnel called on Lou and took him out of class nearly every day to make repairs or troubleshoot problems with everything from simple tasks to wiring and plumbing in the large school he attended. The hired custodian was unable to solve these problems which seemed so easy for my dad. He could also do difficult math problems, however, could not explain how he arrived at the conclusion just having an innate capability to solve problems. So often the explanation was necessary in traditional learning, howbeit, dad was anything but traditional. His approach was simple but unique and he definitely was skilled in a multitude of trades. He had a special ability to view life, it's trials, and challenges alongside opportunities with a keen and uncommon vision. His desire was strong to help not only his family, but others in general and never stopped seeking ways to improve life on every level.

At a very young age, I think when I was 4 years old, my mom became pregnant and into her pregnancy developed severe issues. It was discovered that she was carrying twins and while in the hospital, the doctors found she only had one kidney and considered that possibly as Eleanor grew in her own mother's womb with her twin, only one kidney was formed. Her twin brother, Charles (Butch) later at 80-years-old had to also be on dialysis because he too, only had one kidney and it failed. Two kidneys are not needed to live a normal healthy life, nonetheless, the twins she now carried, coupled with existing high blood pressure put all of their lives and my family life in danger. The twins died and my mom lived although it was a sad time in her and dad's life for a while. She recovered living a busy life full in a small town with her loving husband, children, family and travel. Life was very good.

When I was about 15-years-old, mom, Eleanor, had been ill with what I know now was Strep throat. She was particularly stubborn about seeing doctors, especially after her earlier experience losing her twins and not frequenting doctors as a child. Over a period of about one week, she became increasingly worse and stayed in bed, all day, which was abnormal for this active, vivacious person. I had been checking in on her each day after school and in the evening. About a week into this behavior, I arrived home from school and went into her bedroom to see if she was better. To my alarm, she seemed delirious; almost unconscious. I rushed to see my dad and because of my alarm, he came from work and checked in on her and immediately called an ambulance. He was angry that she was hard headed and unreasonable about doctors.

The ambulance came quickly and rushed to the hospital only 3 miles away, with me accompanying mom in the ambulance. Dad had to finish a bit of work and he came a little later. I was now in the command position in the hospital hallways, elevators, nurses' station, hospital room and standing guard over mom's bed with her breathing shallowly. No one came, nothing was done for two hours or more and suddenly alone with her, she struggled and wanted my hand. Taking her hand, I am faced with a decision to stay or break free and dash to the nurse's station to get help. I went for help. The nurse actually ran back to her room with me, probably seeing the panic in my face and I stayed outside the door and heard a bunch of commotion. Lights blinking along the hallways and I was wondering what the heck was happening as a group of doctor-looking people ran into my mother's room, and a priest tapped me on the shoulder, asking, "Is that your mother?" as he took my hand.

The term, code blue, was unknown to me, during that event and years after it had happened although I was a player in the surreal hospital scene of saving my mom's life that day. The doctors were successful in resuscitating mom and re-starting her heart. That is also the day she had her first of only a few treatments called peritoneal dialysis. This is different than Hemodialysis and was only a temporary "fix" until Eleanor could have a surgery on her wrist called a fistula, to prepare her for hemodialysis treatment so they could "hook up" to the machine.

A fistula, the way I understood it, was necessary due to the 2 large needles used to allow the blood to "hook into" the tubing running into the machine. The opening of the needle had to be large enough to allow enough blood flow out and travel through the tubing into the "filter", which was the workhorse of the cleansing process, and back into the body. Because they were so large, they could not be inserted into a vein, an artery size opening was needed to accommodate the huge needles. If I was squeamish about blood, consider how I felt about blood and huge needles! So, the fistula, somehow, connects the vein and artery together so the vein becomes enlarged enough to allow these needles to be installed. Not so simple in my perspective.

Each time a patient is dialyzed the two huge needles need to be inserted (and later removed). The blood is then pumped around in circles, out of the body into a machine, through the filter of the semipermeable membrane where it is actually cleaned, then back into the body. This circling cycle must be completed about 7 times per treatment. The goal of treatments was to lose weight. Weight loss because it is fluid building up in the bloodstream with toxic waste that the filter removes. Sounds weird, but basically, the patient is weighed before treatment and again after aspiring to lose between 7-12 pounds. This is old information, from my grey matter of dialysis past. I do not know how much weight loss is expected in modern dialysis. Of course, there is more to this process, but that was my first basic understanding. From there, my mom had the few peritoneal treatments, fistula surgery and began her hemodialysis treatments.

Walking out of that dialysis ward at Holy Name Hospital in Teaneck NJ after her first treatment, we all were absorbed in our own thoughts, much I do not remember. The story actually begins here because, on dad's mind was the expense of this treatment and how to keep his wife alive. He had no health insurance on us, and his savings was substantial but limited. The hospital treatments were very expensive, and at the time it was encouraged that the patient/spouse or patient/friend be taught how to administer dialysis at home, purchase their own machine and supplies and by doing so, decrease the cost by half. There was no monetary medical assistance provided by any agency at that time so that is what the majority of the patients did, hurry to train to be on "home-dialysis." Generally, the patients had treatments 3 times a week for 6 hours at a time in those early years. The training for home dialysis usually took 2-3 months, or 24-36 treatments, however, that was traditional and, dad was not traditional. He trained in 5 weeks of treatments, had his "store bought" machine, supplies and area all set up at home in time for mom's 6th week on treatments. The staff at Holy Name were quite impressed and to my knowledge, Lou probably still holds the record.

The things on Lou's mind were myriad, but he had noticed during mom's first hospital treatment that a clamp used on one of the tubes was very difficult to turn and get the correct tightness to adjust the pressure. The nurses had to use a hemostat as if they were a pair of pliers to try to turn it and regulate the pressure of blood flow with much aggravated verbal complaint each time the pressure rose too high or too low making that ungodly alarm squeal. The first night home from his experience, he went into his workshop and did what he always did when he saw that something could be improved and would help make life easier, he began working on a clamp design with a much finer thread and a larger knob so it could be regulated easily with just a person's fingers.

On his second trip back to Holy Name for the treatment, he brought his newly designed and manufactured clamp, and used it. The nurses on staff raved and wanted to know where he got it because they all wanted one! Needless to say, when he got home that night, back to his workshop he went and created enough for the nurses and fellow dialysis patients before the next treatment. This little clamp made life much easier for all of these people and Lou, began to refine the clamps and eventually applied for a patent. He received the patent and named the new piece of medical hardware The Flostat. Our family self-marketed it and sold it to dialysis units across the U.S. at a very low cost. As technology changed in later years, and machines were somewhat altered his hardware become obsolete.

Family routine took on many changes once dialysis entered our lives and from the beginning, it was apparent that mom did not adjust well to being held captive and her appearance and demeanor shifted. She tried most of the time to remain positive and upbeat, but the time spent on hemodialysis was cutting into her fun life. The large dialysis machine, a Travenol RSP, loomed heavy in the living room even when not in use. Her social activities with family dropped off, as did her energy and Eleanor became a shadow of what she once was physically and mentally.

Lou saw the writing on the wall and came terms with his limited time for work and play as well. He decided to sell the family business to his brother and partner for many years so he could spend time with mom and find a way to pursue what they loved to do: travel.

Traveling while on dialysis then was sort of possible, but complicated due to the detail of arrangements and the possible risks involved of dialysis in strange clinics. Clinics were not in abundance in those days as the treatment of Renal failure was still very new in the medical society. Mom disliked the thought of allowing anyone other than her husband to do her treatments and put the needles in her arm.

Lou had time to think as he sat with mom those six hours during treatments 3 times a week. His wife's life was literally in his hands and the stress of that notion lead him to realize they both were in bondage to this machine. He wanted to travel and enjoy the time together, not dread it.

I don't remember exactly when his tinkering mind began to assemble the idea, but it was not long after they started on home dialysis. He was the caregiver, treatment administrator and because of this could not ignore the fact that this manufactured Travenol RSP machine was not designed with the patient or operator in mind. Lou couldn't help himself as he picked it apart and visualized it differently. He realized that the engineers who developed it probably had never put needles in their loved one's arm or sat for 6 hours at a time watching this life-giving transaction of fluids. It was a mere machine to them, just an instrument. As he re-arranged the location of items in his mind while he sat there, once again inspiration came.

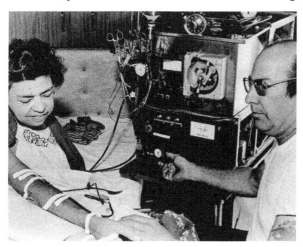

This was not a difficult or complicated machine as far as the mechanics go, he thought. He had all the tools to fabricate a design much smaller and more efficient.

He knew he had to use certain parts of the existing machine, such as the blood pump, as this was highly specialized, but mostly it was just pairing down, and re-arranging things. The frame he fabricated himself, as well as most of the parts he could not readily find in the hardware store. This undertaking had one end-result in mind. Reduce the size, streamlining operation to make it compact and portable for travel in the LouEl, their newer model bus he had finished just before life as they knew it ended, and life on dialysis began.

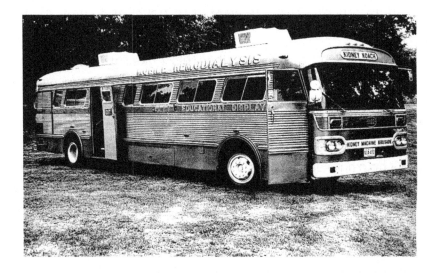

This was a GMC 1955 4104 Greyhound type bus and it remained their favorite. He transformed it into a beautiful living area with upscale Formica, wood flooring, a well-organized kitchen with professionally made cabinets. Everything that they needed was self-contained, including a larger Honda motorcycle for the two of them to explore and investigate the secret places waiting for them. While he dreamed and schemed about the portable machine, he also went about shifting the area in the bedroom of the bus making some changes of layout to house the machine for treatments there. He wanted his wife to have a beautiful view out of the windows to see the spectacular scenery, different each time Eleanor was confined for her life-saving treatment.

The compact machine was carried back and forth by dad from his garage workshop and into the house, as it weighed under 50 pounds. We had a long kitchen table and most of the time it sat at the end so Lou could look at it while he ate breakfast, dinner or just drank coffee pondering the design. The time came for mom to "try it out," and she was totally willing and entirely trusted Lou and his skill set. Lou had the Travenol RSP set up side by side with his more practical compact machine as a back-up plan in case things did not go as intended. The first run on the compact machine was a perfect performance and weight loss on target. The two celebrated, then brainstormed and prepared their escape in the LouEl.

Their trips were unique. I went on the first adventure with them to help as dad dialyzed mom for the first few times in a mobile situation as my brother was newly married and busy with his life. All of their past fun and experience leading up to this point was utilized as dad decided to ask assistance from, at first, the local firemen in the town of our first stop. He also inquired at police stations for support, as well as reached out to many friends they had met. He needed to have a good, pure source of water to hook into, not heavily chlorinated, so he asked for it. In turn, the people who became involved were so responsive and their desire to learn about this subject was aroused. The first stop, in Pennsylvania, the firemen were so interested to see the machine and know what it did that they asked if the local newspaper could stop by during the treatment and interview them. Of course, mom and dad were happy to spread information about dialysis and transplantation, and readily agreed.

From that time on, Lou himself sought out the local papers or news stations in hopes of educating others about the disease and what they could do to help. They both took on this new mission with fervor as it evolved with each stop. Traveling now had a different flavor as they still enjoyed the fun and some of the freedom they once knew, but the purpose of spreading information about dialysis and transplantation was their objective. There are multitudes of news stories and articles from various states written about the home on wheels and dialysis. One summer day, the LouEl was parked on one of the main streets in Boston, MA, and unbeknownst to the passersby on the side walk, Eleanor was receiving a dialysis treatment. They began to feel comfortable enough using their water in the bus and the generator, but dad always had a back-up plan if necessary, never putting mom at risk.

In our many conversations during those days, most of it focused on kidney disease, Lou clearly saw dialysis as a short-term solution while people awaited a transplant. Dialysis was not a way of life, only a temporary, short term solution until the patient had a new kidney. Not all were candidates for such, but the biggest problem was that there were not enough donors. The second biggest being a rejection of the organ, but his focus was on organ donation and what it meant to countless lives and families. While the first kidney transplant was in 1954, information about it was uncommon and Lou was a believer that information lead to understanding.

However foreign this subject was to their lives, Lou was observing that people were open and willing to hear about dialysis and transplants, so he purchased another bus but not to convert into a home, but rather to be emptied as a clean slate. The walls, and ceiling, were updated with modern Formica covering, the floors carpeted with indoor/outdoor carpet to bear up under crowds and soften the atmosphere, and recessed bright lights installed to museum-like conditions. A simple display board was created about the Artificial Kidney and how it worked with the original Travenol RSP machine on exhibit at one end. This new bus was called The Kidney Koach.

Together with my brother and his new wife, they worked to schedule visits of the Kidney Koach at schools and State Fairs around the country using the US postal service and long-distance calling as their means of promotional contact. Using his own money, he formed a non-profit organization called The Kidney Krusade. This display was mostly used to educate young people and answer questions, provide donor cards to those interested, but on several occasions, he used it in conjunction with fundraising events to help sponsor a dialysis patient in need of funds to continue dialysis. In those early days, as I stated, there was no assistance from agencies. In 1972 legislation was passed that provided federal government financing for nearly all Americans with kidney failure. Until that legislation was activated, however, many people were in need.

Lou was in contact with the National Kidney Foundation that was founded only 6 short years before our family became part of kidney disease statics and with the Ruth Gottscho Kidney Foundation, having on several occasions met with Eva Gottscho. Although fundraising and helping people in their immediate circumstances was important, he was convinced that in the "long haul" a better solution for a better life was needed and available. Education and focus were the key to developing the answer and it was doable. Up Until 1960, Kidney disease was considered fatal, but with the advent of dialysis, now reduced to just a chronic disease. Quite a milestone!

Lou continued to modify his design and created a total of 3 completed compact machines, all used by Eleanor and all worked perfectly. Mom's nephrologist, Dr. Robert Rigolosi, was more than a physician to our family and of course, he had somewhat of a celebrity as patients, plural, since Lou and El were inseparable more now than ever. He had invited us to attend a medical convention at the Palmer House Hotel in Chicago. It was an eye-opening experience for me, and I loved the different instruments, medical machines, and hardware being displayed as well as the lectures by doctors from all over the U.S., most way out of my league of understanding at age 16. Our doctor invited many of the attendees to visit our family's home on wheels and view dad's compact dialysis machine built for travel. We had permission to park the bus, the LouEl, right on the street in front of the Palmer House for 2 hours for attendees to participate in the extension of the items on display.

In each model of the machine dad designed from the first, he uniquely mounted the blood pump to the front of the machine. All manufactured machines to that point had the blood pump mounted on the top; every brand basically in the same place. When dad moved the pump to the front, it was because he wanted his wife to be involved in the dialysis process sustaining her life, so she would not feel helpless. Get the patients involved in their health and treatment! The emotional side of dialysis is another long story in and of itself. She could monitor it easily on the front and see if there was a problem immediately.

After the Chicago convention ended there was one company that marketed a new machine on its heels: it was called Sarns. Dad saw an advertisement for this new design by Sarns and noticed that the blood pump was prominently mounted on the front of this newest model, just like his own. Lou did not accept it as coincidence but was pleased and complimented by this action and he wrote to the owner of the company who he knew was in the LouEl that day in Chicago mentioning the new position of the pump. Mr. Sarns answered Lou's letter confirming he had used dad's idea and sent him a brand new Sarns blood pump for him to use on his next design, a gift in the monetary value of at least a thousand dollars. Every dialysis machine I see now, the blood pump is mounted on the front. This seems a small thing, but to me represents Lou Hamilton, cutting edge functional designer of dialysis machinery.

When Eleanor died in August of 1973 in our home in Ohio, I was 17 years old. We had moved to Ohio in hopes of her getting a kidney transplant as the waiting list was very long in the populated surrounding area of New York City where we lived my entire life. He chose a small town outside of Columbus, because after the painstaking, time intensive research Lou did again by US postal service, he found that the percentage of transplant to the number on the waiting list was optimal there. He sold our family home that he and mom built themselves right after I was born, and we moved my senior year of high school.

When we had first moved into the home we bought there, Lou and El missed their friends and activities of their New Jersey life, but stayed close and did not travel far hoping to have a phone call once El was on "the list", the transplant list. They finally decided to take the LouEl and go back to Jersey for a visit after many months of waiting and longing for a visit. They were only there a few days and my brother, and I received a phone call saying they had a kidney match for her. We leaked the word to the doctor calling that they were in New Jersey and he thought we did not actually live in Ohio and he was about to pass mom by for the next person on the waiting list who matched.

Lou got a hold of him on the phone and said he and mom would arrive at the hospital very soon, whenever the doctor needed them to be there, they would arrive. Lou's best friend in New Jersey gave him some cash, a ride to the airport and he rented a Lear Jet and flew back to Columbus, arriving there even before the other recipient from Dayton Ohio arrived. Lou was one to be prepared, and he brought his portable machine with them on the jet. While at the hospital, and awaiting to be prepped for surgery, they learned that the donor's kidneys were too damaged in the car accident to be used for transplant. Very disappointed we all drove to our home south of

Columbus. Lou set up the machine he brought home with them, and the next day mom dialyzed at home. Flight reservations were made with a commercial plane to return to the LouEl in New Jersey the day after her treatment. Even in 1972 Lou and Eleanor Hamilton traveled with a portable compact Hemodialysis machine weighing under 50 pounds on a commercial airline stowing it inside the cabin.

A man who dropped out of the eighth grade self-made a medical dialysis machine, designed, developed and manufactured 3 of these compact, portable machines, patented a clamp used in dialysis and began a non-profit organization building a bus display promoting information throughout the United States, while administering dialysis to his wife 3 times a week. All of this in only 3 ½ years. Even to me, his daughter, after all these years, I am awe struck thinking of his accomplishments in such a short time with limited funds and under difficult circumstances.

As life moved forward when mom died, I was not involved in anything about dialysis, nor did I pursue it. I really wanted to forget about it. I seldom ever saw or heard mention of it on TV or movies in the 45 years mom has been gone. While cleaning out some items one day in 2017, I found some pictures of a film the US government made of our family called Dialysis on Wheels in 1972.

The "film" had recently been found by my brother on YouTube Historic films and I was inspired to post this link and a few of the picture's dad took as they filmed it to a Facebook site concerning my old hometown, Waldwick NJ. I had never posted on that site before. Later that day I was contacted by a person with a non-profit organization called 1 in 9. A friend of hers was from Waldwick, even though she and her husband resided in Phoenix AZ, and he saw the post I put up. She and I spoke for at least an hour or two and I was astonished to learn that although I have been removed from dialysis all these 44 years (in 2017), that much was still the SAME concerning dialysis machines and procedure with little advancement or change.

Everything that I heard and observed was not so new to me. Kidney disease as usual, only more widespread, and not the alternatives for a better life that Lou had envisioned. Granted, the machines were more modern, compact, tightly contained and sleeker than the original Travenol RSP, mom's first machine in 1970, howbeit, many still live lives, a limited life in more than one sense of the word, dependent upon a machine. Lou often said, "Dialysis is not a way of life, but a necessary stepping stone to a better, easier life." Dialysis is NOT A CURE. Kidney disease is now in 8th place, killing and destroying more families than breast cancer and prostate cancer but is relatively unheard of by the general public.

There is a better way. The time is now. There is a "cure". Someone or a collective someone is out there with inspiration to be cutting edge and the fuel that is needed to propel technology into a new era, focus and direction. Let's put some of these dreams up on the kitchen table and view them with a renewed hope, not just sustaining life, but making life better moving forward downstream. New designs and inventions are out there trying to find you. Be fearless. Are you listening?

Written for Lou and Eleanor Hamilton and their vision of love for you.

Pioneering the Future

Elizabeth Saladin, MD

Stories passed down from generation to generation; stories about the good old days. Growing up in a family with mixed cultures and backgrounds, I recall the different stories. On my mother's side, Native American stories about the Creator and lessons from animals and mother Earth is meant to teach us respect and to pass down wisdom. On the other hand, as early as I can remember from my father's European background were stories of pioneering inventions and futuristic endeavors that impacted people and changed lives. His dad, my grandpa, lived right next door to us; he and I had a special bond. He was inspirational to me and because of his accomplishments and belief that nothing was impossible. I never had an idea that was too big.

Grandpa's house was filled with years of memories and objects collected from all over the United States. However, there was one thing that always captured my curiosity. In the corner was something very special to my grandpa and he always loved talking about. As a child, I thought everyone had a small dialysis machine in the living room. Grandpa's stories reminded me of Frankenstein. I mean, this machine kept my grandmother alive! He loved to tell me all about my grandmother. Unfortunately, I never knew her.

Eleanor Hamilton was my grandmother. She was only 44. She was born in 1929 and she was a twin. She married my grandpa in 1949, and they had two kids, my dad, Lou Jr and my aunt Maryjane. Their life seemed like an action movie to me. Stories of travel and adventure, motorcycles and Indy 500 races created excitement and likely instilled in me a confidence in my own future endeavors and adventures that I would not have even imagined as a child. Unfortunately, she was diagnosed with renal failure in her early 40's. It was believed she suffered from post-streptococcal glomerulonephritis, a complication from a streptococcal infection. Later, it was discovered that she was born with only one kidney, which made fighting this battle extra challenging.

Ultimately, my grandmother, Eleanor required lifesaving treatments of hemodialysis 6 hours 3 times a week. In the 1970's this was usually done in a hospital setting and cost about $36,000 a year, most times paid for out of pocket by the patient and family. My grandfather owned a small Lawn and Garden business in NJ and thankfully was able to pay for this to keep his wife alive. After reality set in and 'Eleanor Hamilton' became a name on a kidney donation recipient list, my grandfather became consumed with the desire to overcome this. He studied the dialysis machines that she was dependent on and after only a few treatments in the hospital my grandfather purchased a machine and began home dialysis. But this was not enough. Determined to return to life on the road, he drafted ideas and dreamed of a way to design such a machine that would fit on their family bus/converted mobile home.

Now, bear in mind, my grandpa only had an 8th-grade education. Amazingly he created a machine ¼ the size, that was able to be stowed and operated within the family's bus.

When it came time to try the new kidney machine on grandma the first time, my dad remembers Dr. Rigolosi at the Holy Name Hospital in Teaneck, NJ suggesting they try it out on the dog first! Everyone laughed, and I cannot imagine the tension in the room or the trust that my grandmother must have had in my grandfather to attempt hemodialysis on the first small portable dialysis machine.

To everyone's amazement, it worked! Eleanor fared well, and the machine got the approval of the doctor and technicians. They were no longer restricted from travel! For 3.5 years my grandmother's life was prolonged, but more importantly, her quality of life was preserved. She lived her life to the fullest until the very end. I hear that she loved to sing. She was funny and free-spirited. She was kind and loving, and I was always told of how much she would have spoiled me if she had been given the opportunity to know her grandchildren.

My dad tells of the night they got a call from the transplant surgeon that a donor's kidney was available; I see the sadness in his eyes and hear it in his voice. He initially speaks with excitement as he called his mom and dad who were, guess what…traveling! They were in another state, and he urgently explained they had to get home now! My grandpa hired a private Lear jet, and with a police escort, they were there the next morning. Sadly, the donor's organs were unable to be transplanted due to injury resulting from trauma. It was so close. They did all they could to increase the likeliness of getting a kidney. My grandparents moved their residence to Ohio after they researched that more kidney transplants were done in this state than in their home state. My grandfather also sold his business to fund this noble cause. This is a story of love.

During the time grandma was on dialysis, my family, including my mother, embarked on a mission of public awareness called the "Kidney Krusade." They converted another bus into a mobile educational display that gave the public an overview of kidney disease and treatment options. They displayed the kidney dialysis machine and explained how it worked, and more importantly they encouraged people to become organ donors. Although my parents had only been married for one year my mom still speaks of love and admiration for Eleanor. Mom was also very committed to the Kidney Krusade and lived on the bus with my dad for a whole year traveling the

U.S. Aft er a few years of visiting schools, fairs, and community events they were able to reach over 200,000 people that toured the "Kidney Koach," and amazingly 60,000 people became documented organ donors. People all over were amazed. Documentaries, newspaper articles, and TV interviews are evidence today of what an impact the Hamilton's made. Sadly, Eleanor passed away due to complications of renal failure in 1973.

At 18, I left home and married my high school sweetheart. He believed in my dreams as much as my grandpa did and he was willing to do whatever it took to make sure I would be successful. I knew I had a passion for the medical field and helping people but I was not prepared for how far that would take me. I honestly cannot explain what came over me to even have the thought of becoming a doctor. Health professionals were in my family; my mother a licensed medical technician, a sister who is a pharmacist and another a pharmacy technician, but physicians there were none. My grandpa's health soon declined early in my college years. He never got to see me graduate from medical school, although I proudly shared his story and documentaries every time I could throughout medical school and residency.

No, I did not become a nephrologist, although I have the utmost respect for this specialty. Instead, I found my love in Family Medicine. I can care for people of all ages, and my focus is that of preventing disease. I get to meet people where they are along this life's journey, and if I am lucky, I get to play a small part in helping to make a life with good health. I also have a calling to use my education and background to contribute and help improve the health of Native people. I was able to attend medical school through a scholarship through the Indian Health Service, and I have a deep, personal commitment that extends beyond my service requirements of the program. I was honored to work for the Eastern Band of Cherokee Indians in Cherokee, NC for four years following residency and later moved home to Oklahoma and currently work for the Absentee Shawnee Tribe.

Diabetes and hypertension are prevalent in alarming rates in the Native population, which often leads to kidney disease. Every day I have the opportunity to encourage patients to create healthy lifestyles and help them find ways to maintain control over the disease, not letting the disease control them. We use all available tools to screen for diseases and have dedicated nephrologists who travel to our rural clinics to see our patients. Thankfully the rates of chronic kidney disease in Native populations are declining due to the increased screening and interventions and patient efforts.

Growing up, I felt like I was a product of two different worlds. I wasn't sure where my place was, who I was. I was not sure how they connected, whom I would become. Looking back, I am grateful for both of my parents' cultures and the way they molded me into who I am today. I give God the glory for the things He has done in my life, and I look forward to how He will continue to use me during my time on this Earth. Thank you for allowing me to share my story.

I look forward to sharing these stories with my two daughters as they grow up and find their own place in this world.

On the Road With 1in9

Analyn Scott

Towards the end of 2016 I was inspired to take 1in9 on the road to bring awareness and capture more stories from across the United States for our documentary, so in March of 2017, our family hit the road on a 35' RV for our nearly month-long East Coast tour and epic adventure.

We had Raymond's dialysis machine with about 5 days of treatments on board, and had additional supplies strategically shipped to specified locations along the way. Raymond and I would take turns driving as we made our way from Phoenix to: Dallas, Nashville, Atlanta, Charleston, Charlotte, Richmond, D.C., Baltimore, NYC, Cleveland, Chicago, St. Louis, Albuquerque, and back home to Phoenix.

In June of 2017, we embarked on our West Coast Tour, traveling from Phoenix to: Tucson, Southern CA, Los Angeles, San Jose, Oakland, San Francisco, Salt Lake City, and home to Phoenix for a few weeks before heading back to Dallas, TX where we had a booth at MegaFest.

As you can imagine, all of this was quite an adventure for our family. Raymond and I still jokingly debate over which was more challenging: (1) My driving a 35' RV through Manhattan and Harlem, or (2) His having to drive through a severe thunderstorm and tornado warning through Oklahoma with nowhere to stop, having to drive 30 mph for over 6 hours.

We met so many wonderful people from all walks of life throughout our journey, and regardless of what region, state, city, community or neighborhood that we visited, we witnessed several common needs and trends.

Lack of awareness is a HUGE issue everywhere, but it was still shocking to hear so many medical and/or dialysis professionals referencing how many people are "crashing" into dialysis. Many of which had clues in their medical records and lab results that were never explained to them. Over and over this was validated with the patient stories we were hearing first hand. Far too many people we spoke with that had diabetes and/or high blood pressure were not aware of the fact that those are the two leading causes of kidney disease.

Also, many dialysis patients and/or their family members we met were not aware that home dialysis was even an option for them.

We hosted an event in Harlem during our RV tour in March 2017 and there were several people that asked us if we would please come back, that there was a major need for awareness in their community. Of course, we would, only next time we would fly! Discussions began right away with our friends at ImageNation Cinema Foundation to collaborate and return during one of their Summer Festival outdoor film screenings that August.

Earlier that summer a friend and former client of mine from my I.T. days, Steve from NJ, sent me a link to "Dialysis on Wheels 1972", a historic film following Lou and Eleanor Hamilton. His message to me was, "the folks who it's about were/are from my home town!" Their story amazed me, and I reached out to their daughter Maryjane, who had posted the video. As we shared our stories with one another, I'll never forget Maryjane's shocked response to learning that most people on dialysis do so in-center. She couldn't understand how her father was able to make her mother a travel-sized dialysis machine over 45 years earlier, and yet most people were now being tethered to a larger machine in a dialysis center.

Our conversation sparked a renewed interest for Maryjane to pick up where she left off as a teenager and partner with 1in9 to raise awareness and keep her parent's legacy alive. When I mentioned joining us at our upcoming event in Harlem, Maryjane was all-in!

It was surreal for us all to see the dialysis machine her father Lou Hamilton made in 1972 for her mother Eleanor next to Raymond's home dialysis machine at the 1in9, *"What's Really Goin' On,"* panel discussion in Harlem. It was an eye opening and empowering experience for the community as well. The majority of the attendees had family or friends on dialysis yet we're completely unaware of the option and benefits of home dialysis.

Fate would have it that the night of this event also marked the 44th anniversary of Eleanor Hamilton's passing at the young age of 44, but the legacy she and Lou created together lives on.

I echo Maryjane's call to usher in a new era for kidney disease. As our collective drum beat grows louder, let it beckon others with passion and vision like Lou Hamilton to step forward with their unique piece of the puzzle to a cure.

PART 8:

Getting to the Root

Discover Your Microvascular Health. Improve Your Future

By Gary Hennerberg
Part 8 © Microvascular Health Solutions

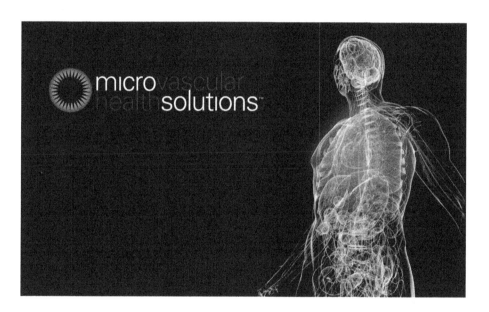

Microvascular.com | GlycoCheck.com

Kidney Health and Hope from a New Discovery

If you haven't heard of the glycocalyx, you're not alone. Even many medical professionals aren't aware of its importance to good health because glycocalyx research is a new emerging science from the scientific community. It's now being introduced to medical schools, and gradually being shared with the general public.

The glycocalyx is a micro-thin protective gel layer that lines the inside of all blood vessels throughout your body, including your kidneys and other vital organs.

In this chapter, you'll learn the history and back story of how the glycocalyx was discovered, scientific research studies from more than 65 hospitals and research centers worldwide (as of early 2019), and the solution that can improve glycocalyx and kidney health.

The bottom line news is this: a weakened glycocalyx begins a spiral that is linked to kidney disease along with several other diseases and conditions.

So how do you know if you have a weakened glycocalyx? It could be that your body is signaling you with early warning signs that you're chalking up to aging. But if you want to definitively know, some healthcare practitioners offer a simple, non-invasive test where a video microscope camera measures blood flow in small blood vessels under the tongue to reveal if you're on the brink of health problems. A low score reveals that your glycocalyx is weak and that your organs might be at risk and already comprised.

Thankfully, this story is only beginning. There is hope for the future from a new, easy-to-take all-natural dietary therapeutic that doesn't require a visit to your doctor, a test, or a prescription.

A 5,000-Mile Journey

The journey to these breakthroughs in glycocalyx research and a new solution begins with two people, 5,000 miles apart living in two separate continents.

Robert "Bob" Long is a successful businessman who lives in Utah. The journey that lead Bob to establish a new company began in an unpleasant way—with a health scare in 2009 when he was 54 years old, had Type 2 diabetes, and

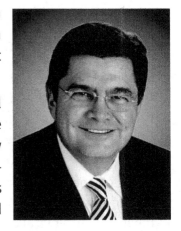

was 65 pounds overweight. The stresses of a life constantly on the road, building an international company, and the pressure to always perform at his job as a top sales executive led him to pause when he noticed a recurring tightness and pain in his chest.

He went to his personal physician who did a basic check and was concerned that he was at risk for a heart attack and suggested he immediately go see his friend who is a cardiologist. So, the doctor made a quick call and sent Bob to the regional medical center to meet with a cardiologist who was working there that day.

A one-hour morning appointment dragged into the evening. The assumption after performing several tests and confirming that he hadn't had a heart attack was that Bob had a blockage in the arteries of his heart which was causing the tightness he felt when he walked up hills. So, the doctor recommended that he perform an angiogram with the intent of putting in stents if they found any blockages to prevent a heart attack in the future.

Good News and Bad News

But after the test, when the doctor showed Bob and his wife the results, he said, "I have good news, and I have bad news."

"Give me the good news first," said Bob.

"You haven't had a heart attack, so there's no damage, and there isn't any major blockage that required a stent," replied the cardiologist.

"So, what's the bad news?"

"We don't really know what's causing your chest pain and tightness. All I can do is prescribe some medications, suggest you change your lifestyle, lose some weight, and start exercising. Come back in 30 days and we'll do a follow-up."

"I Should Have Lived a Better Life."

Like most patients, what Bob heard and thought to himself was: "Dude! You really screwed up! You should have lived a better life. You don't have much time left. And the doctors don't know how to help me."

The doctor started writing a stack of prescriptions. Bob researched what each was supposed to do, but each one had significant side effects. He said to himself, "I don't want to take these drugs for the rest of my life! The side effects that they each list sound worse than my fear of what's wrong!"

As timing would have it, Bob had just been part of the sale of a company he had helped grow so he had financial resources, and perhaps more importantly, time on his hands. Since his doctor couldn't tell him what was wrong with him, Bob decided to take his health into his own hands and figure it out for himself. Bob started to exercise, lost weight, and 30 days later had somewhat better stats, so his doctor told him he was on the right track, reduced the drugs and told Bob to come back a year later for a follow-up.

Fast forward one year. Bob had a stress EKG test to check again for blockage. The result: Bob looked fine, all is normal. Still no answers. But Bob was motivated to do something. He could have gone home, taken the pills from the doctor, lived a crappy life, and surrendered, but that wasn't the path Bob chose to take.

A Quest to Discover the "Why"

Bob has always believed that there is a reason for everything. He embraced that his greater purpose in his life was to find out the "why" behind what starts a downward health spiral and to see if there is a solution that could help millions of people including himself.

By chance—well, perhaps it wasn't by chance, but part of God's plan—a good friend's brother, a physician, told Bob the news of research about the glycocalyx and its composition. Upon hearing how the glycocalyx lines every artery, vein, and capillary, and how the primary composition of the gel-like glycocalyx is similar to some compounds found in certain seaweeds, a light turned on. What if the health of his glycocalyx could be his problem and if natural ingredients could be the solution?

Diet had always been on Bob's mind as a possible culprit. Seaweed is not part of most North American's diet and culture. Yet seaweed is packed with vitamins, minerals, and antioxidants and it turns out the same type of compounds found in the structure of the glycocalyx.

It's no secret that people from Japan and the Mediterranean live longer than people who live in North America. Seaweed makes up an important part of the diet in Japan. And in the Mediterranean, where smaller farms grow more of their own fruits, vegetables, grapes, olives, and artichokes using organic methods, people in that region of the world enjoy better health.

But the solution isn't just to eat seaweed, more vegetables, and more fruit. It's very difficult to eat enough of these foods daily. Let's face it. A balanced diet is much more than seaweed, vegetables and fruit. Unfortunately, many people consume pre-prepared processed foods. Most households simply can't afford the cost of buying a high volume of fresh organic produce, even if they were available to purchase.

Bob hired a biochemist, nutritionist, and seaweed experts. He was determined to become an expert himself in nutrition to discover if his theory that diet was linked to glycocalyx health was accurate. To learn more about the glycocalyx, he set up an alert on Google so that any time a paper was published about the glycocalyx, he would know it.

An Alert That Forged a New Partnership

As Bob began to read publicly available glycocalyx research, he noticed a name that kept recurring as a thought leader. Bob thought to himself, "Someday I'd like to meet Dr. Hans Vink and have him answer my questions one-on-one." Dr. Vink lived in the Netherlands, some 5,000 miles away from Bob's home in Utah.

Then one day in early 2012, Bob got an alert about a patent that had been issued to Dr. Vink for a glycocalyx testing device that had been referenced in earlier papers that Bob had been reading. Dr. Vink had been studying the glycocalyx since the 1980s, but it took until the mid-1990s for technology to enable peering deep inside the capillaries to take pictures.

After the discovery of a very thick glycocalyx, and development of new techniques to take the early pictures, it took another decade of research to see if glycocalyx health was linked to diseases and conditions. Out of necessity, Dr. Vink created a glycocalyx testing device, with the first version of this device patented in 2012. By this time, Dr. Vink had been established as a glycocalyx expert worldwide.

So nearly a half world apart, Bob and Dr. Vink were both on a parallel journey to learn about the glycocalyx. While Dr. Vink was researching the importance of the glycocalyx for vascular health and organ function, Bob was testing glycocalyx nutritional ingredients on himself.

What Bob didn't have was a way to confirm if the dietary therapeutic he was testing on himself was making a difference. He needed, and desired deeply, to confirm that he was on the right path. Dr. Vink held the keys to that part of this story with his newly patented testing device.

A Glycocalyx Research Pioneer

Dr. Vink may technically be considered a biomedical researcher. More specifically, he is a pioneer in the study of the endothelial glycocalyx. He is one of the first researchers to study the glycocalyx when he focused his expertise on medical imaging. As a result, Dr. Vink and his team were one of the first research groups to capture realistic images of the glycocalyx and focus on its significance.

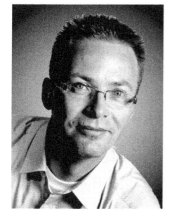

Dr. Vink developed the testing technology system to clinically assess the glycocalyx. He is often sought out to lecture at universities and medical institutions around the world due to his expertise in the science of glycocalyx observation and his passion for sharing his extensive understanding of the vascular system. Dr. Vink earned a PhD in Medical Physics from the University of Amsterdam in 1994, where he began his study of the glycocalyx. He continued his research as a postdoctoral fellow at the University of Virginia and returned to Amsterdam in 1997 to continue his work. He was awarded a Research Fellowship from the Royal Netherlands Academy of Arts and Sciences for his study of the glycocalyx from 2000 through 2005.

In 2005 he became an Established Investigator of the Netherlands Heart Foundation. In 2006 he joined the department of Physiology at Maastricht University, where he continues glycocalyx research within the Cardiovascular Research Institute Maastricht (CARIM).

Breakthrough: A Clinical Test of Glycocalyx Health

The technology that allows testing the glycocalyx is a system known today as GlycoCheck™. This revolutionary patented imaging software and hardware system includes a small video microscope camera placed under the tongue to measure a key aspect of the overall health of the glycocalyx. Dr. Vink learned that testing under the tongue provides a representation of the entire body's glycocalyx health and its impact on microvascular health.

In 2012, when Dr. Vink secured a patent on the first generation of GlycoCheck, and Bob became aware of its existence, Bob wasn't quite sure how to approach Dr. Vink. Bob was concerned that because he didn't have any research or medical credentials, Dr. Vink wouldn't take his inquiry seriously. But Bob was determined after taking his first generation dietary therapeutic to get tested, and he didn't want Dr. Vink to know he was making himself a guinea pig with his own formula.

Bob had an idea. As mentioned earlier, he was working with a biochemist who was helping to formulate his therapeutic. She was going to a science meeting in Switzerland and France so Bob asked her a favor: would she please contact Dr. Vink and arrange a meeting with him in the Netherlands and ask to be tested on his new GlycoCheck device. She did. Part of Bob's plan was that since she wasn't taking the therapeutic yet, her test could serve as a baseline. If the discussion with Dr. Vink went well, she could make an introduction to Bob. She met for an entire day with Dr. Vink, was tested, and told him that she wanted to have Bob Long contact him about his research.

Within a day, Bob emailed Dr. Vink, telling him he had read all of his papers and was a big fan, and asked if he could meet with him in the Netherlands. Dr. Vink was surprised to find out that Bob had read his papers and was well versed in the research. A few weeks later, Bob was in Dr. Vink's office to be tested on the GlycoCheck device.

Bob deliberately didn't tell Dr. Vink he was taking his therapeutic. Bob had theorized specific ingredients would improve glycocalyx health, so he had his scientific team formulate his first-generation product. They had started a double-blind study to test if the therapeutic was making a positive impact at the dose they hypothesized would work.

Still, Bob was a bit nervous to find out if all his time and money developing a therapeutic would produce a better test outcome. Dr. Vink, in the meantime, thought to himself that Bob surely wouldn't have a healthy glycocalyx. Bob was overweight and had Type 2 Diabetes, and Bob suspected he had compromised the glycocalyx in the arteries of his heart.

Burgers and Fries

Dr. Vink knew his glycocalyx was healthy because he tested himself on many occasions. He was thin, had a healthy diet, and exercised regularly, so he showed Bob what a healthy score would look like.

"You Americans like your burgers and fries," Dr. Vink kindly told Bob, hoping not to disappoint him. "So, I don't expect you'll have a good score."

Dr. Vink measured Bob on the GlycoCheck. It only takes a few minutes to calculate the results. Moments later, Dr. Vink said "let's measure you again." Bob couldn't tell by the reaction if that was good or bad. A few moments passed by, and Dr. Vink turned to a colleague sitting next to him, started speaking in Dutch, and pointed to the screen. Bob had no idea what they were saying.

"Will I live or die?" Bob asked. After all, earlier in the day Dr. Vink had shown Bob several studies he had conducted. One of those studies was on sepsis patients in ICU that had shown the GlycoCheck system accurately predicted who would live, and who would die, if the Glycocalyx was not restored quickly.

Dr. Vink replied, "I wanted to test you twice because I'm confused. Your score is better than mine, and I didn't expect that with your medical history."

"I Cheat"

Bob jokingly said, "I cheat."

"What do you mean you cheat?"

"I have been developing a therapeutic and taking it for several months. My reason for coming here to meet you, and get tested, was to see if I my formulation was working."

During this same meeting, the scientist who met Dr. Vink months earlier had her glycocalyx health measured again. After the return from her first trip and test months earlier, she started to take Bob's therapeutic. She was tested again, and her score had improved markedly.

"My reason for traveling 5,000 miles to meet you and get tested was to see if I was on the right track," said Bob.

The "So What?" Discovery

At that moment, Dr. Vink's eyes teared up and he began to become emotional.

"Do you realize you might be on the path to discover the 'so what'?" said Dr. Vink. "In the 25 years I've worked to prove the glycocalyx is real, I had to develop the testing device. When I performed the test for people, and when they have an unhealthy score, their immediate question has been 'what can I do to improve my score?' And all I could do was give them the typical answers: lose weight, eat better, exercise, don't smoke, and so on. I've never had a true solution I could offer."

Hoping this might be the outcome of his test, Bob brought along samples of the therapeutic he had developed and gave some to Hans (by now, they were on a first name basis). Hans took some right of way, and the next day when they got together again, Hans tested himself, and he was surprised to see that his score had improved.

Career Crossroads: Answering the "So What?"

Hans told Bob that he didn't know of any drugs, supplements, or other therapeutics on the market that specifically supported glycocalyx health. Now Hans was out of his comfort zone. Would he make the career decision to remain a pure academic researcher mostly focused on publishing papers and getting grants? Or would he dedicate himself to translational glycocalyx research with a mission toward bringing this knowledge to the world to measure people's glycocalyx health? And would Hans join Bob to figure out the rest of the 'so what?' that could be a life-changing improvement in people's health and longevity?

During that meeting, Bob and Hans decided to work and form a company together. The explicit purpose was to improve the GlycoCheck technology and develop a test score that could be easily understood by both healthcare practitioners and patients. A big part of their work together has been to test multiple compounds in the therapeutics' formulation to isolate how those ingredients would affect physiology and the body's reaction. They tested themselves and other volunteers and ultimately developed the formula that is now known as Endocalyx™. That formula was so unique that they were granted a patent for the method of treating the glycocalyx by the US patent office in 2018.

In the years since, Dr. Hans Vink has published, or co-authored, over 200 peer-reviewed research papers about the glycocalyx. In 2018 alone, there were 13 peer-reviewed papers published using the GlycoCheck as a tool to understand the development and progression of multiple diseases. In addition, about 9,000 other papers by other researchers have cited Dr. Vink's work.

This is only the first part of the extensive story about the glycocalyx. In the next section, you'll learn more about its role, how it works, why it's important to good kidney health, and the Endocalyx therapeutic that is helping people with multiple conditions and diseases return to better health.

Glycocalyx Science, Early Warning Signs, and the Solution

Microvascular research has either been ignored or overlooked for years. Mostly because the microvascular system—the capillaries—have been hard to study and see. But that's changing.

Research conducted by Dr. Hans Vink, PhD, as featured previously, reveals how he had been studying the microvascular system since the 1980s. It wasn't until the mid-1990s that technology advancements enabled peering deep inside the capillaries to take pictures. The discovery of a very thick glycocalyx, and development of new techniques to take the early pictures, has led to ongoing research to determine how a compromised glycocalyx is linked to diseases and conditions.

Pictures and videos from inside the capillaries reveal the presence of the endothelial glycocalyx. It's a vast protective gel lining that touches each of your trillions of cells. Every cell of your body is nourished by the blood that travels through the capillaries that make up 99% of your circulatory system from head to toe.

Placed end-to-end, scientists estimate the body's capillaries would extend over 60,000 miles, enough to go around the earth two and a half times. Is it any wonder they've been overlooked? It's in this 99% of our circulatory system where essential organ nutrition takes place, and when it breaks down, it leads to a downward health spiral.

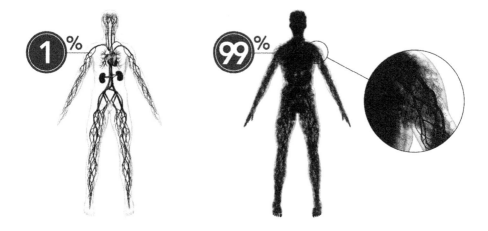

Inside the capillaries every heartbeat delivers vital nutrients and oxygen, while waste is removed from each cell. This essential exchange of nutrients, oxygen, and waste removal becomes less efficient with aging, poor diet, lack of exercise, genetics, stress, and smoking.

More Than Hollow Tubes

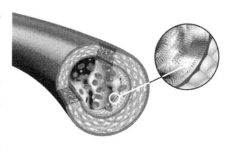

In the past, blood vessels were thought to be simple hollow tubes. But with today's high-resolution video microscope cameras, the discovery of the glycocalyx reveals that the entire circulatory system is coated with a gel-like lining that protects the inside walls of the arteries, veins, and capillaries. Its integrity is essential to the healthy function of all the cells, organs and body systems.

The glycocalyx keeps your body healthy in three critical ways.

First, it functions as the natural trigger that stimulates the production of nitric oxide. Nitric oxide is vital in controlling blood flow and blood pressure. The glycocalyx stores anti-oxidants and, working together with nitric oxide, both increase blood flow, on demand, when organs call for it. For example, when you're walking upstairs. Or even when your brain is working through a difficult problem. Bottom line: your body needs a thick and healthy glycocalyx to efficiently regulate blood flow.

Second, a healthy glycocalyx allows your body to engage more of the available capillaries of the microvascular system when blood flow increases. This is critical to regulate the supply of nutrients and oxygen, and the removal of waste and carbon dioxide, according to the body's level of activity, such as when you exercise. Bottom line: While blood flow control is important, the glycocalyx allows your body to engage more capillaries when organs demand nourishment and waste removal.

Third, capillaries are much more than simple hollow tubes. In fact, their inner surface is coated with a non-stick glycocalyx that prevents loss of capillaries through fluid leakage, blood clotting and inflammation. This coating helps to prevent cholesterol and fat from leaking and sticking, and it keeps blood clotting and inflammation under control. For example, when your body's healthy, it can repair a simple cut or fight an infection. Bottom line: a healthy glycocalyx not only engages more capillaries when blood flow goes up, but it also protects the capillary network and even the entire vascular system from deterioration and loss.

Ongoing clinical research from more than 65 hospital and university research studies confirms that a compromised glycocalyx and a damaged microvascular system are linked to organ starvation.

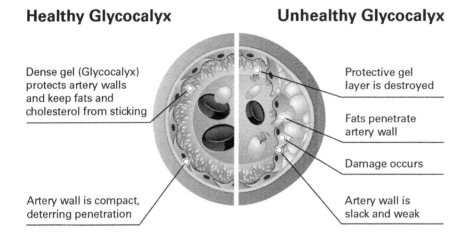

Healthy Glycocalyx
- Dense gel (Glycocalyx) protects artery walls and keep fats and cholesterol from sticking
- Artery wall is compact, deterring penetration

Unhealthy Glycocalyx
- Protective gel layer is destroyed
- Fats penetrate artery wall
- Damage occurs
- Artery wall is slack and weak

Kidney Disease and Other Conditions Linked to Microvascular Health

Looks can be deceptive. You may look—and even feel—healthy on the outside, but inside your microvascular system, a completely different situation could be developing. Your organs may be starving from the lack of nutrients and oxygen and weakened by waste that has accumulated and isn't removed. Organ starvation is one reason that diseases begin in the body.

There are several diseases and conditions linked to poor microvascular health:

Kidney Disease (impaired production of urine causing increased blood volume and hypertension). Vascular link:

- Damage of micro vessels causes leakage of blood proteins into urinary space, damage of renal filtration units and kidney failure. (See references at the end of this chapter for more detail).

Diabetes (high blood glucose level). Vascular links:

- A healthy microvascular system is important for transport of glucose from blood to organs.

- High blood glucose damages the microvascular system and causes blindness, kidney failure, heart attack and stroke.

Hypertension (blood pressure is higher than accepted level). Vascular links:
- Hypertension is associated with loss of microvascular density.
- Hypertension increases cardiovascular risk (heart attack, stroke, kidney failure).

Heart Disease (loss of pump function of heart). Vascular links:
- Loss of microvascular density causes heart attack.
- Insufficient number of capillaries per heart muscle fiber impairs heart pump function (heart failure).

Stroke (blood clot in brain artery causing brain damage). Vascular links:
- Damage to vascular wall causes blood clots.
- Microvascular damage causes White Matter Lesions with poor neurological prognosis.

Dementia (early cognition impairment: neurological complication). Vascular link:
- Healthy microvascular system is essential to maintain intact neuro-vascular unit and support normal neurological function.

Septic Shock (loss of circulation blood volume causes drops in blood pressure, impaired organ blood flow resulting in acute kidney failure, reduced lung function, heart attack, stroke and brain damage). Vascular links:
- Leaky micro vessels result in loss of blood plasma volume to tissue space.

- Damaged vascular wall causes increased blood clotting and inflammation.

Inflammatory Disorders (rheumatoid arthritis, vasculitis, allergies, glomerulonephritis, autoimmune diseases, scleroderma and atherosclerosis). Vascular links:

- Attack of microvascular system by inflammatory cells results in loss of capillaries.
- Increased capillary permeability causes tissue edema.

Cancer (uncontrolled growth of tumors). Vascular link:

- Leaky micro vessels allow tumor cells to enter the vascular system and redistribute to different parts of our body, causing tumor metastasis (secondary tumors).

How Organ Starvation Begins

Your organs are healthy when they are nourished with vital nutrients and oxygen, and when waste and carbon dioxide are removed.

Every heartbeat is an opportunity for replenishment. This replenishment—an exchange of nutrients and waste removal—takes place in the capillaries of the microvascular system.

When organs starve, it sets off several stages of a downward spiral:

1. Over time, aging, poor diet, lack of exercise, genetics, stress, smoking—and even conditions such as diabetes and high blood pressure—combined with other risk factors, degrade the gel-like lining of the blood vessels.

2. Damaged micro vessels (capillaries) become leaky, lose function and the number of capillaries decreases. Early warning signs begin (read more about those early warning signs later in this chapter).

3. Vital delivery of nutrients, hormones, and oxygen and removal of waste and carbon dioxide is compromised.
4. Organ starvation worsens, weakening vital processes in the heart, kidneys, lungs and brain.
5. Diseases can set in, including:

- **Kidney Disease**
- **Heart Disease**
- **Lung Disease**
- **Stroke & Dementia**
- **Septic Shock**
- **Inflammatory Disorders**
- **Cancer Metastasis**

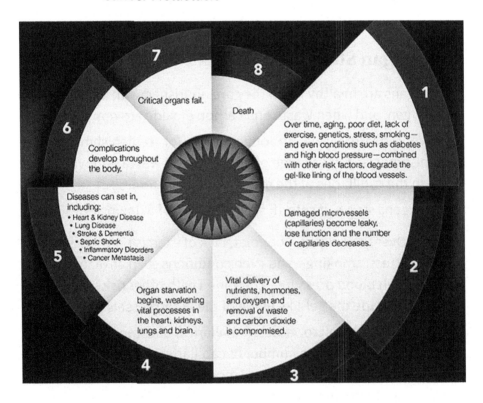

6. Complications develop throughout the body.
7. Critical organs fail
8. Death

Watch the downward spiral video at Microvascular.com.

Early Warning Signs

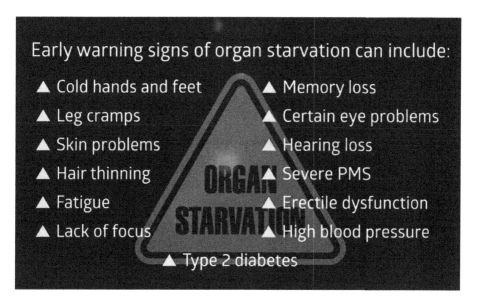

Early warning signs of organ starvation can include:

- Cold hands and feet
- Leg cramps
- Skin problems
- Hair thinning
- Fatigue
- Lack of focus
- Memory loss
- Certain eye problems

- Hearing loss
- Severe PMS
- Erectile dysfunction
- High blood pressure
- Type 2 diabetes

All these early warning signs could be caused your glycocalyx breaking down inside your microscopic capillaries.

Watch the video about the early warning signs at Microvascular.com.

Research and Proof

As of this writing in early 2019, some 65 hospitals and universities around the world are using GlycoCheck to study diseases and conditions. Those projects include research on:

- Kidney failure and Hemodialysis
- Type 2 Diabetes
- Stroke
- Early Cognition Impairment
- Epilepsy
- Syndrome X
- Pre-eclampsia / HELLP
- Sepsis / Septic Shock
- Pre-eclampsia
- Atherosclerosis
- Heart failure
- Premature Atherosclerosis
- Malaria / Dengue
- Obesity / Fat disorders
- ESRD Proteinuria
- Inflammation

The list of worldwide hospitals and universities, along with diseases and conditions being studied, continues to grow.

Studies are being conducted in Africa, Asia, Australia, China, Europe, Japan, Russia, and the United States. Below is a sample of a few hospitals and universities:

- Mayo Clinic
- Duke University
- University of Pittsburgh Medical Center
- VA Hospital of Salt Lake City
- Arizona State University
- University of Utah
- Wayne State University
- University of Michigan
- University of Iowa
- Children's Hospital in Philadelphia
- University of Oxford
- Harvard Beth Israel
- Leiden University Medical Centre
- Copenhagen Steno Diabetes Center
- University of Exeter
- Shanghai University
- University of Tasmania
- Juntendo University Emergency and Disaster Medicine, Tokyo
- Nanyang Technological University

Dozens more, along with new additions, can be viewed at GlycoCheck.com.

Expanding GlycoCheck Testing Availability

As mentioned previously, you can get an overall health score with GlycoCheck, a patented technology, and the test can be easily performed in a healthcare practitioner's office.

In 2019, GlycoCheck is being introduced in medical and healthcare practitioner's offices throughout North America. GlycoCheck testing is available from healthcare practitioners who are part of the nationwide *Healthy U Rx* and *Rx 2 Live* networks, along with other independent healthcare offices.

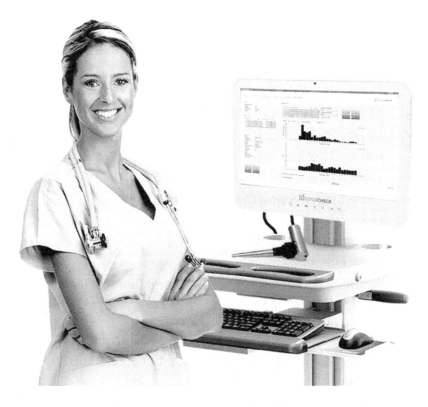

GlycoCheck gives you and your healthcare provider the one single number—a MicroVascular Health Score™—that alerts you when trouble could be lurking deep inside your capillaries.

The good news is that even if you have a poor score, you can easily improve your health.

GlycoCheck works by simply placing a video camera microscope under the tongue for a few moments to video record, analyze, and objectively report a single, overall, MicroVascular Health Score™. GlycoCheck counts the number of blood vessels and capillaries and measures red blood cell concentration. It also measures flow rate, and if and how deeply the blood cells penetrate into the protective glycocalyx gel lining—a sign of deterioration.

Each test includes a baseline score and video of the microvascular blood flow and tracks how, over time, the microvascular score declines with health deterioration, or improves by taking a specifically formulated therapeutic that support glycocalyx health.

Watch the video about GlycoCheck at GlycoCheck.com.

GlycoCheck Methodology

The GlycoCheck video microscope camera detects the erythrocytes within the small, sublingual blood vessels. Then, the GlycoCheck software records, detects, and analyzes the blood vessels ranging from 5 to 25 micrometers in diameter.

The automatic analysis consists of the detection of the center lumen of every blood vessel and detection of the outer boundaries of the erythrocytes. The distance between the red blood cell column and this outer boundary is identified as the perfused boundary region (PBR). The PBR value is calculated on 3,000 individual positions, which makes the measurement results sensitive, yet very reproducible. A higher PBR value corresponds with a proportional decrease in the thickness of the glycocalyx layer.

Reversing a Compromised Microvascular System

Fortunately, you can reverse a low MicroVascular Health Score with a patented proprietary dietary therapeutic that has been clinically shown to repair and improve the health of the glycocalyx. This patented proprietary formula is a blend of synergistic ingredients. It's called Endocalyx™.

The ingredients are sourced from regions around the world where people are known to live longer and live healthy active lives.

Endocalyx is made from concentrated extracts of seven natural ingredients. These ingredients contain the same compounds that make up and protect the structure of the glycocalyx. It's a specific blend, right down to the molecular structure that makes all the difference in the result of taking Endocalyx daily.

This patented combination of ingredients, in specific dosage amounts, stimulate three actions that restore, rejuvenate, and protect your glycocalyx and microvascular system.

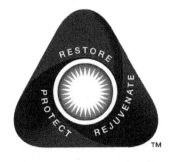

Restore: The first result of this specific blend comes from polysaccharides that restore the protective structure of the glycocalyx and enables repair of the glycocalyx matrix. Polysaccharides are long sugar chains that can interact with proteins and other molecules of the glycocalyx to restore its protective structure.

Rejuvenate: The second result comes from the amino sugars, the precursor for polysaccharide biosynthesis that rejuvenates your body's ability to produce more of the glycocalyx protective gel. Amino sugars enable the cells of the vessel wall to produce more glycocalyx polysaccharides and rejuvenate the body's ability to produce more of the protective gel.

Protect: And the third result comes from antioxidants that protect the polysaccharides of the glycocalyx from breaking down.

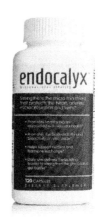

Scientific research backs up that these synergistic ingredients, when combined together, deliver these vital results in your microvascular system.

As Endocalyx strengthens the glycocalyx, the blood in your entire vascular system is better able to reach and energize each cell of your body. Then all the cells of your body, including your kidneys, brain, heart, and muscles, are amply supplied with oxygen and nutrients.* This means that more blood cells, carrying more nutrients and vital oxygen to all of your muscle, skin, and nerve cells, restore warmth, feeling and comfort.*

As Endocalyx strengthens the glycocalyx, it helps optimize the structure of the capillaries. From head to toe, optimal capillary function delivers many benefits, including clearer thinking, increased energy, improved performance, more youthful appearance, and greater comfort.*

The better each brain cell is supplied with oxygen and nutrients, the better your mood, the clearer your mind, the more productive your thinking.*

Healthy skin, hair, and eyes depend on a steady supply of oxygen and nutrients to renew, grow, and stay healthy.* Skin color and tone are enhanced.* Your hair and nails are stronger and healthier.* And, your eyes are clearer and brighter.*

Watch the video about Endocalyx at Microvascular.com. Endocalyx is available at Microvascular.com.

> *These statements have not been evaluated by the Food and Drug Administration. This product is not intended to diagnose, treat, cure or prevent any disease.

Discover Your Microvascular Health
and Improve Your Future

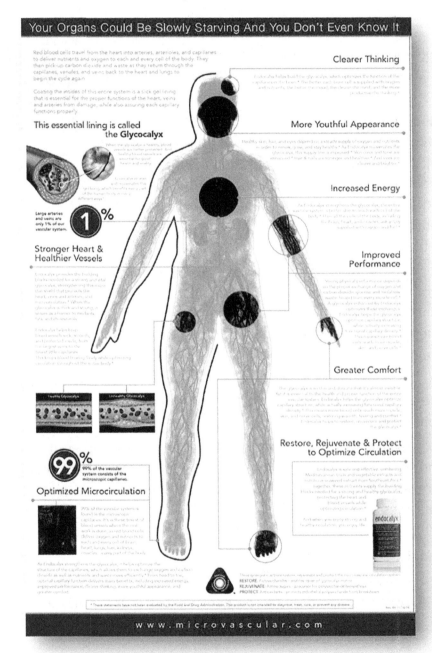

Published Papers

For reference, below you'll find a few published papers related to kidney disease and vascular health. Additional published papers can be read at GlycoCheck.com or Microvascular.com.

Association of kidney function with changes in the endothelial surface layer.

https://www.ncbi.nlm.nih.gov/pubmed/24458084

Dane MJ[1], Khairoun M, Lee DH, van den Berg BM, Eskens BJ, Boels MG, van Teeffelen JW, Rops AL, van der Vlag J, van Zonneveld AJ, Reinders ME, Vink H, Rabelink TJ.

[1] Author information: Department of Nephrology, Einthoven Laboratory for Vascular Medicine, Leiden University Medical Center, Leiden, The Netherlands; †Department of Physiology, Maastricht University Medical Center, Maastricht, The Netherlands, ‡Department of Nephrology, Nijmegen Centre for Molecular Life Sciences, Radboud University Nijmegen Medical Centre, Nijmegen, The Netherlands.

Abstract

BACKGROUND AND OBJECTIVES:

ESRD is accompanied by endothelial dysfunction. Because the endothelial glycocalyx (endothelial surface layer) governs interactions between flowing blood and the vessel wall, perturbation could influence disease progression. This study used a novel noninvasive sidestream-darkfield imaging method, which measures the accessibility of red blood cells to the endothelial surface layer in the microcirculation (perfused boundary region), to investigate whether renal function is associated with endothelial surface layer dimensions.

Design, Setting, Participants, & Measurements:

Perfused boundary region was measured in control participants (n=10), patients with ESRD (n=23), participants with normal kidney function after successful living donor kidney transplantation (n=12), and patients who developed interstitial fibrosis/tubular atrophy after kidney transplantation (n=10). In addition, the endothelial activation marker angiopoietin-2 and shed endothelial surface layer components syndecan-1 and soluble thrombomodulin were measured using ELISA.

Results:

Compared with healthy controls (1.82 ± 0.16 μm), ESRD patients had a larger perfused boundary region (+0.23; 95% confidence interval, 0.46 to <0.01; P<0.05), which signifies loss of endothelial surface layer dimensions. This large perfused boundary region was accompanied by higher circulating levels of syndecan-1 (+57.71; 95% confidence interval, 17.38 to 98.04; P<0.01) and soluble thrombomodulin (+12.88; 95% confidence interval, 0.29 to 25.46; P<0.001). After successful transplantation, the perfused boundary region was indistinguishable from healthy controls (without elevated levels of soluble thrombomodulin or syndecan-1). In contrast, however, patients who developed interstitial fibrosis and tubular atrophy showed a large perfused boundary region (+0.36; 95% confidence interval, 0.09 to 0.63; P<0.01) and higher levels of endothelial activation markers. In addition, a significant correlation between perfused boundary region, angiopoietin-2, and eGFR was observed (perfused boundary region versus GFR: Spearman's ρ=0.31; P<0.05; perfused boundary region versus angiopoietin-2: Spearman's ρ=-0.33; P<0.05).

Conclusion:

Reduced renal function is strongly associated with low endothelial surface layer dimensions. After successful kidney transplantation, the endothelial surface layer is indistinguishable from control.

Damage of the endothelial glycocalyx in dialysis patients.

https://www.ncbi.nlm.nih.gov/pubmed/23085635

Vlahu CA[1], Lemkes BA, Struijk DG, Koopman MG, Krediet RT, Vink H.

[1] Author information: Division of Nephrology, Department of Medicine, Academic Medical Center, A01-132, Meibergdreef 9, 1105 AZ Amsterdam, The Netherlands.

Abstract

Damage to the endothelial glycocalyx, which helps maintain vascular homeostasis, heightens the sensitivity of the vasculature to atherogenic stimuli. Patients with renal failure have endothelial dysfunction and increased risk for cardiovascular morbidity and mortality, but the state of the endothelial glycocalyx in these patients is unknown. Here, we used Sidestream Darkfield imaging to detect changes in glycocalyx dimension in dialysis patients and healthy controls from in vivo recordings of the sublingual microcirculation. Dialysis patients had increased perfused boundary region and perfused diameters, consistent with deeper penetration of erythrocytes into glycocalyx, indicating a loss of glycocalyx barrier properties. These patients also had higher serum levels of the glycocalyx constituents hyaluronan and syndecan-1 and increased hyaluronidase activity, suggesting the shedding of these components. Loss of residual renal function had no influence on the imaging parameters but did associate with greater shedding of hyaluronan in blood. Furthermore, patients with higher levels of inflammation had more significant damage to the glycocalyx barrier. In conclusion, these data suggest that dialysis patients have an impaired glycocalyx barrier and shed its constituents into blood, likely contributing to the sustained endothelial cell activation observed in ESRD.

Acute ischemic injury to the renal microvasculature in human kidney transplantation.

https://www.ncbi.nlm.nih.gov/pubmed/20810613

Snoeijs MG[1], Vink H, Voesten N, Christiaans MH, Daemen JW, Peppelenbosch AG, Tordoir JH, Peutz-Kootstra CJ, Buurman WA, Schurink GW, van Heurn LW.

[1] Author information: Dept. of Surgery, Maastricht Univ. Medical Center, PO Box 5800, 6202 AZ Maastricht, The Netherlands

Abstract

Increased understanding of the pathophysiology of ischemic acute kidney injury in renal transplantation may lead to novel therapies that improve early graft function. Therefore, we studied the renal microcirculation in ischemically injured kidneys from donors after cardiac death (DCD) and in living donor kidneys with minimal ischemia. During transplant surgery, peritubular capillaries were visualized by sidestream darkfield imaging. Despite a profound reduction in creatinine clearance, total renovascular resistance of DCD kidneys was similar to that of living donor kidneys. In contrast, renal microvascular perfusion in the early reperfusion period was 42% lower in DCD kidneys compared with living donor kidneys, which was accounted for by smaller blood vessel diameters in DCD kidneys. Furthermore, DCD kidneys were characterized by smaller red blood cell exclusion zones in peritubular capillaries and by greater production of syndecan-1 and heparan sulfate (main constituents of the endothelial glycocalyx) compared with living donor kidneys, providing strong evidence for glycocalyx degradation in these kidneys. We conclude that renal ischemia and reperfusion is associated with reduced capillary blood flow and loss of glycocalyx integrity. These findings form the basis for development of novel interventions to prevent ischemic acute kidney injury.

An extensive list of current published papers can be read at GlycoCheck.com or Microvascular.com.

A Gift from Heaven

Analyn Scott

Saturday January 30, 2016 was a bittersweet day for our family, one that would set events in motion that would alter the course of our lives in a very unexpected way. We received the call from my mom that afternoon that my grandmother had passed. Raymond and I moved forward with our dinner plans to celebrate our 17th wedding anniversary, reminiscing about fond memories over dinner.

My great-aunt, who I had not seen in years, approached me at the family luncheon in Utah following my grandmother's funeral February 6, 2016 and said, "Analyn, aren't you doing something with kidneys?"

"Yes", and before I could say anything further, she said, "Come with me," walked Raymond and I over to a table and said, "this is my son Bob." "Bob, this is your cousin Analyn." Then she walked away. Alright, my only clue to why she pulled us to meet Bob was kidneys, so I started to explain who we were and our connection to kidney disease. "Oh, I get it", he said. "I'm Bob Long, CEO of Microvascular Health Solutions and we've come up with an all-natural dietary therapeutic that is helping people improve their kidneys, high blood pressure and diabetes."

I'll be honest, I didn't have much hope for it to improve Raymond's kidneys because he had been on dialysis for so long, but my interest was piqued to learn more about how this might help improve his high blood pressure and diabetes. As we shared more about Raymond's health, I could see Bob's interest level increasing too, as he explained more about the glycocalyx, and asked if he could meet with us the next day to administer a GlycoCheck™ exam, curious to see what Raymond's microvascular health score would be.

We were eager for Bob to arrive to the home we were staying at in Park City the next day to perform the GlycoCheck test on Raymond. My mom, Raymond and I were all mesmerized by the origin story, science, clinical studies, and testimonies Bob shared about the GlycoCheck and therapeutic when he sat down with us. Logically and in my gut, I knew that this was a major missing link that could help get to the root of so many medical conditions that impact kidneys.

We all hovered around the laptop as Raymond placed the GlycoCheck device under his tongue and video of his capillaries appeared on the screen. Despite trying 3 times, Bob was not able to get any readings on Raymond. He then tested my mom and me, and sure enough the machine was working fine. I remember Bob's eyes getting big and a look of concern came across his face before saying, "I've never not been able to get a reading on anyone." Then said, "Here, take these," as he handed Raymond five months' supply of Endocalyx™, the microvascular therapeutic that Bob had formulated to improve Raymond's glycocalyx health, so he could get started on right away.

After Bob left, I gazed out the window at the beautiful snowy mountains that surrounded us, and I felt an intense sense of gratitude. I excused myself and retreated to our guest room bathroom and wept. It was one of the most spiritual experiences of my life. I wept for my grandmother and had such an overwhelming feeling of gratitude that she had given us a gift from heaven. I just knew that it was going to have a significant impact for Raymond and others, but I never could have predicted what was about to unfold.

If you're keeping track of dates from Chapter One, you may have noticed that this was just a few weeks before Raymond performed at the Dancing with The Stars AZ gala, which took place February

20, 2016. The six months of dance practice helped him get in great physical shape, as you could see in the picture, I shared in Chapter One. Raymond was on 3 blood pressure medications at the time and had been on insulin daily for over 14 years. Following his performance at the gala, Raymond's dance shoes were set aside, and he went back to his normal exercise routine. Endocalyx was the only thing that was new. This gives us a great baseline to start with.

Within two weeks of Raymond taking Endocalyx, he noticed that his blood pressure was getting lower. He continued to monitor every day and kept his nephrologist aware of the changes he was experiencing. Within about two months his nephrologist took him off one of his blood pressure medications. Over the course of about 8 or 9 months, he was able to continue taking Raymond off the remaining blood pressure medications one by one, and his readings were averaging between 110/70 to 120/80, without any blood pressure medications. This was amazing! Even with all his medications, Raymond was never able to maintain pressures this good.

Within four months Raymond was off all insulin and is not on any diabetic medication at all! After a couple of years of taking Endocalyx, his latest A1C was 5.6, which is excellent.

The early morning hours of Memorial Day 2016, Raymond developed a fever, so we followed our protocol, packed his bag and headed to the Phoenix VA Hospital ER department. It appeared to be pneumonia, so he was admitted to the hospital. Later that morning his breathing was getting worse, so they put him on low oxygen. Shortly afterwards Senator John McCain came in to Raymond's room, as one of his stops to visit Veteran's and thank them for their service.

As the day progressed so did the difficulty breathing and Raymond was equipped with an oxygen mask to increase the flow of oxygen, but by that evening it was getting worse. Additionally, his blood work came back showing that the staph infection he was recently treated for had bounced back. The Dr. started him on antibiotics and suggested they move him into the ICU, sedate and intubate him with a breathing tube proactively now so they wouldn't have to do so in an emergency situation. This was all new to us. Raymond had been in the hospital multiple times over the years for pneumonia, but never had struggles breathing like this. We both agreed, not fully understanding what all of this meant, but trusting that it was best to stay ahead of whatever was going on.

I wasn't fully prepared to see Raymond on the breathing machine, sedated, and hooked up to all the tubes and monitors. The next morning his blood pressures were scary low. Raymond's liver levels were declining, but thankfully quickly improved. The dialysis tech was able to wheel the dialysis machine to his bedside to continue with the necessary treatments. I stayed alert and on top of everything that was taking place. I prayed, others prayed, and I had an inner peace knowing that Raymond was going to make a full recovery.

Raymond was intubated on a Monday evening and was taken off the machines Thursday afternoon. When they brought him out of sedation, they let Raymond know he couldn't talk for a few hours to protect his vocal chords, so they gave him a clipboard with paper and pen to write any questions he had. One of the first questions he wrote was to ask what day it was. When I told him Thursday, he had a look of amazement and disbelief. In fact, he then wrote down THURSDAY??? Last he remembered it was Monday and later said he had no awareness of time during his ordeal.

The kids were so excited to see Raymond that Thursday, and his face lit up when he saw them. I didn't want them to see him while on all the machines and I tried to keep them encouraged that dad was going to be fine, but I knew they were worried. They were still a little apprehensive, but once they put on some cartoons to laugh together,

I could see the fear finally dissipate and they too knew that all was going to be well.

The picture above shows Raymond on Friday walking the halls of the hospital. His doctors were amazed at how well and how quickly he had recovered from being so sick. The kids were with family and I was helping Raymond settle into his new hospital room out of the ICU. I put on some hospital socks, arranged some hospital snacks, and had him scoot over so I could get comfortable next to him in the hospital bed for us to watch a movie together before I would head home for the night. One of the nurses came in to bring a new pitcher of water She looked over, smiled and said, "He looks so great for being septic." WHAT?? Turns out Raymond did not have pneumonia after all, he had severe sepsis and respiratory failure!

With this knowledge, I was able to do some research and see that the signs of sepsis were there, that at the time I had no idea Raymond's body was fighting valiantly against. Maybe the doctors assumed I knew, or that someone else had told me, either way I see it as a blessing and believe in a way I was being protected too.

According to *sepsis.org*, sepsis and septic shock can result from an infection anywhere in the body, such as pneumonia, influenza, or urinary tract infections. Worldwide, one-third of people who develop sepsis die. Many who do survive are left with life-changing effects, such as post-traumatic stress disorder (PTSD), chronic pain and fatigue, organ dysfunction (organs don't work properly) and/or amputations.

According to the CDC, anyone can get sepsis from an infection, but the risk is higher in: People with weakened immune systems, babies and very young children, elderly people, people with chronic illnesses, such as diabetes, AIDS, cancer, and kidney or liver disease, and people suffering from a severe burn or wound.

As I was discussing all of this with my mom, she reminded me that this sounded similar to one of the clinical studies Bob had shared with us where they had performed GylcoCheck tests on patients in ICU settings with sepsis/septic shock and could predict which patients would live and which patients would die based on their Microvascular Health Score™ (MVHS). Thinking back to just 4 months earlier, knowing that Bob couldn't even get a reading on Raymond to tell him what his MVHS was, it sunk in just how big my grandmother's gift was. Had Raymond not been taking Endocalyx to help regenerate his glycocalyx and improve his microvascular system I don't believe he would still be alive.

While still recovering in the VA hospital the news hit that Muhammad Ali had died Friday June 3rd, 2016 from septic shock in another local hospital. My heart went out to his family, and I remember thinking how grateful I was that both Muhammad Ali and Raymond were in two separate valley hospitals so they both could have the top ICU medical teams attending to each of their needs. My mind couldn't help to think about the miracle we experienced, and how it was our duty to help share this missing link solution with others so they could have an extra edge in their fight for life.

Raymond made a full recovery and continued to see additional improvements in his microvascular health over time. He previously had not been eligible for another transplant because he had stenosis, or the narrowing of a major artery that would lead to a transplanted kidney. Witnessing the turnaround of Raymond's other vascular conditions, I was curious to see if there was any change in this area, so Raymond scheduled some vascular testing to be re-evaluated. Those results revealed that they no longer saw any stenosis and the blood was free-flowing through that artery. That cleared him from a vascular stand point.

Raymond often looks down at his legs in amazement, seeing thin ankles and veins in his legs and feet that he has not seen in years and continues to take Endocalyx daily.

We've also witnessed improvements in the health of others with whom we have shared Endocalyx. My mom being one of them. In May of 2016 her GFR was 50 (stage 3a), seeing what was happening with Raymond she began taking Endocalyx in September of 2016. She had her blood-work done for her 6-month checkup in November of 2016 and her GFR improved to 79, a "significant increase" according to her doctor.

Several people have shared that since taking Endocalyx, they have experienced improvements in their blood pressures, others with their blood sugars, neuropathy, wounds, cholesterol, and GFR as well. I would get calls and reports back from people saying that they were able to work closely with their doctors and avoid having to start taking cholesterol medication, or that their doctors were able to reduce or remove them from cholesterol and other medications. One, a friend who is on dialysis, was happy to report that under doctor supervision, was able to come off of 3 blood pressure medications. Another friend, a cancer survivor, shared that her kidneys had been damaged from the chemo and medications to the point that her doctors were starting to talk about dialysis options. She was able to turn that around and improve her GFR and kidney function back to stage 3 and avoid dialysis.

I believe this is a major missing link in the fight against kidney disease, and I'm happy to report that we will be launching a 1in9 Microvascular Study, allowing us to pay Grandma's gift forward and positively impact and save even more lives!

PART 9

Lift Up Your Voice

"Armed with knowledge and hope we raise our voices, and collectively we can and will change the trajectory of kidney disease."

Analyn Scott

Here are some ways you can help *Amplify the Sound of Change*:
* Share your "1in9" story at www.1in9Tribe.com
* Like & Share www.facebook.com/1in9KidneyChallenge
* Make a tax-deductible donation at www.1in9Tribe.com
* Start a *1in9 Tribe* Book Club and/or purchase extra copies for family and friends

Microvascular Health Solutions cares about people with kidney disease, and extends a special offer for supporters of 1in9 and readers of this book. Go to 1in9Tribe.com/MVHS to learn more about how you can get tested on **GlycoCheck** and order **Endocalyx**.

For "The 1 IN 9"

There is a silence that must be heard
A diagnostic truth that leaves too many without words.
Though I've been enlisted in this number,
Kidney Disease is a plight we can conquer.
I will not be defined by parenthetical lines
That attempt to confine my mission to reach, "The 1 IN 9".
As long as I live, my Love for Life remains real,
For my Tomorrow's have Dates,
Divine Design has allowed me to make.

And Embodied within this Ocean of Time
Is the strength and resilience of my mind!
So, the world may witness and clearly see,
There is no regretful fear in me.
And the Analysis of Dialysis shall Not imprison
My Dreams with paralysis.

Yes, there are days when treatment forces a fight,
Then I look into the feelings inside caring eyes,
and they invigorate my might.
To be there for my loving family drives me,
And places my Will on Determination's top shelf,
Pity is a struggle I refuse to be felt.

For "The 1 IN 9" ~ Zemill

We understand the realities of our maladies,
Yet we will Trust in Never Giving Up!
With a quickening pace must we promote this race!
For the ones we hold so close in our hearts
And those unknowing souls whose journeys has yet to start.

Because of you that have helped and joined our quest,
The Torch of Hope shall be without rest.
The Spirit of Belief with an unyielding voice,
Will deliver knowledge, care and wisdom
So that millions may Rejoice!
For those who gave and for the ones who give,
You are the Beacon of Possibilities that enables our Message to Live.

And when we all stand at the podium
Of Graciousness and Charity
Your name will be sewn,
Within the tapestry of this narrative.
As one who chose to Rise Up,
To aid the Courage of Kindness to Triumphantly Shine
A euphoric illuminating Light of Relevance Upon "The 1 IN 9"!

Zemill
Copyright 2016 Lyrics Unlimited Publishing

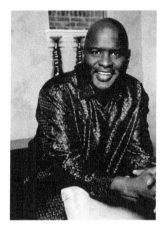 Zemill is a Dallas native who is an award-winning Spoken Word Artist, Performer, Author, and Lyricist. He has performed for the Two-Time Emmy Award Winning Civil Rights Concert hosted by The Black Academy of Arts and Letters! His work has been featured in the U. S., Europe, Canada, and Nigeria. He is one of the most versatile performers on the scene today. He has fused Smooth Jazz, Smooth R&B, Neo Soul and Spoken Word to create his own unique brand of music known as *"The PoJazz Experience."* His new Book *Love Unleashed The Fire And Passion Of Poetry*, his CD *"Timeless,"* and, Newly Released CD *Intimate Pleasures* are destined to be a Mind Engaging Journey and Mellow Music Lovers Favorites!

Bibliography

Part 3: Out of the Shadows: Inspiring a Legacy of Change

1. "ANNOUNCEMENT: PRESTIGIOUS, DYNAMIC ARIZONA PASTOR DIES - BISHOP ALEXIS A. THOMAS," January 19, 2018, http://www.pilgrimway.com/assets/files/Bishop_pressrelease.pdf

Part 4: It Takes a Village

Crowned for Change:

1. National Kidney Foundation, s.v. "Acute Kidney Injury," accessed January 6, 2019, https://www.kidney.org/atoz/content/AcuteKidneyInjury
2. National Kidney Foundation, s.v. "Chronic Kidney Disease," accessed January 6, 2019, https://www.kidney.org/atoz/content/about-chronic-kidney-disease

Slow It Down CKD

1. Mayo Clinic, s.v. "Early signs of chronic kidney disease," accessed January 6, 2019, https://www.mayoclinic.org/diseases-conditions/chronic-kidney-disease/symptoms-causes/syc-20354521

Part 5: Medical Tribe

Vantage Point: A Nephrologist's View of Kidney Disease

1. USRDS 2018 Annual Report, Chapter 5: Acute Kidney Injury, https://www.usrds.org/2018/view/v1_05.aspx
2. *USRDS 2013 Annual Data Report: Table 1.f (Volume 2) Page 430 Analytical Methods*

3. American Journal of Medicine, *AM J Med 2007, Outcomes in patients with CKD referred late to a nephrologist*
4. USRDS 2016 Annual Report, Volume 2, Chapter 1: Incidence, Prevalence, Patient Characteristics, and Treatment Modalities https://www.usrds.org/2016/view/v2_01.aspx
5. NIDDK, https://www.niddk.nih.gov/health-information/health-statistics/kidney-disease

I Am Not My Disease

1. NIDDK, https://www.niddk.nih.gov/health-information/kidney-disease/acquired-cystic-kidney-disease

Part 6: The Drumbeat for Regenerative Medicine

1. David Mogollon, "1in9 Kidney Challenge Founders Visit UA Nephrology Faculty, Researchers, University of Arizona Department of Medicine," May 24, 2017, https://deptmedicine.arizona.edu/news/2017/1in9-kidney-challenge-founders-visit-ua-nephrology-faculty-researchers
2. Cynthia Ritter, "1in9 Kidney Awareness Documentary Visits Division of Nephrology," April 4, 2017, Washington University School of Medicine in St. Louis, Division of Nephrology, https://nephrology.wustl.edu/1in9-kidney-awareness-documentary-visits-division-nephrology/

Part 7: The Wheels of Change

1. https://www.holyname.org/physician/details.asp?phyid=00271
2. 1972 Video: https://youtu.be/TSniabEw-R0

Part 8: Getting to the Root
Discover Your Microvascular Health. Improve Your Future

1. microvascular.com
2. GlycoCheck.com
3. Association of kidney function with changes in the endothelial surface layer: https://www.ncbi.nlm.nih.gov/pubmed/24458084; Dane MJ[1], Khairoun M, Lee DH, van den Berg BM, Eskens BJ, Boels MG, van Teeffelen JW, Rops AL, van der Vlag J, van Zonneveld AJ, Reinders ME, Vink H, Rabelink TJ; [1] Author information: Department of Nephrology, Einthoven Laboratory for Vascular Medicine, Leiden University Medical Center, Leiden, The Netherlands; †Department of Physiology, Maastricht University Medical Center, Maastricht, The Netherlands, ‡Department of Nephrology, Nijmegen Centre for Molecular Life Sciences, Radboud University Nijmegen Medical Centre, Nijmegen, The Netherlands.
4. Damage of the endothelial glycocalyx in dialysis patients: https://www.ncbi.nlm.nih.gov/pubmed/23085635; Vlahu CA[1], Lemkes BA, Struijk DG, Koopman MG, Krediet RT, Vink H.; [1] Author information: Division of Nephrology, Department of Medicine, Academic Medical Center, A01-132, Meibergdreef 9, 1105 AZ Amsterdam, The Netherlands.
5. Acute ischemic injury to the renal microvasculature in human kidney transplantation: https://www.ncbi.nlm.nih.gov/pubmed/20810613, Snoeijs MG[1], Vink H, Voesten N, Christiaans MH, Daemen JW, Peppelenbosch AG, Tordoir JH, Peutz-Kootstra CJ, Buurman WA, Schurink GW, van Heurn LW; [1]Author information: Dept. of Surgery, Maastricht Univ. Medical Center, PO Box 5800, 6202 AZ Maastricht, The Netherlands

Part 9: Lift Up Your Voice

1. Zemill, For "The 1 in 9," Copyright 2016 Lyrics Unlimited Publishing; https://youtu.be/vwq15jkBe1w
2. www.1in9Tribe.com